Patient-centred Communication

LANGUAGE AT WORK

Series Editors: Jo Angouri, *University of Warwick, UK* and Rebecca Piekkari, *Aalto University Business School, Finland*

Language at Work is a new series designed to bring together scholars interested in workplace research. The modern workplace has changed significantly in recent years. The international nature of business activities and the increasing rate of mobility around the world create a new challenging environment for individuals and organisations alike. The advancements in technology have reshaped the ways employees collaborate at the interface of linguistic, national and professional borders. The complex linguistic landscape also results in new challenges for health care systems and legal settings. This and other phenomena around the world of work have attracted significant interest; it is still common however for relevant research to remain within clear disciplinary and methodological boundaries.

The series aims to create space for exchange of ideas and dialogue and seeks to explore issues related to power, leadership, politics, teamwork, culture, ideology, identity, decision making and motivation across a diverse range of contexts, including corporate, health care and institutional settings. *Language at Work* welcomes mixed methods research and it will be of interest to researchers in linguistics, international management, organisation studies, sociology, medical sociology and decision sciences.

All books in this series are externally peer-reviewed.

Full details of all the books in this series and of all our other publications can be found on http://www.multilingual-matters.com, or by writing to Multilingual Matters, St Nicholas House, 31–34 High Street, Bristol, BS1 2AW, UK.

LANGUAGE AT WORK: 5

Patient-centred Communication

Discourse of In-home Medical Consultations for Older Adults

Kayo Kondo

MULTILINGUAL MATTERS
Bristol • Jackson

DOI https://doi.org/10.21832/KONDO5881
Library of Congress Cataloging in Publication Data
A catalog record for this book is available from the Library of Congress.
Names: Kondo, Kayo, author.
Title: Patient-centred Communication: Discourse of In-home Medical Consultations for Older Adults/Kayo Kondo.
Description: Bristol; Jackson: Multilingual Matters, [2022] | Series: Language at Work: 5 | Includes bibliographical references. | Summary: "This book presents a comprehensive analysis of the use of patient-/person-centred communication in providing health care for ageing populations through an ethnographic approach to physician in-home medical consultations in Tokyo, Japan, alongside interviews with physicians"—Provided by publisher.
Identifiers: LCCN 2022016603 (print) | LCCN 2022016604 (ebook) | ISBN 9781800415881 (hardback) | ISBN 9781800415898 (pdf) | ISBN 9781800415904 (epub) Subjects: LCSH: Physician and patient—Japan. | Communication in medicine—Japan. | Patient-centered health care—Japan.
Classification: LCC R727.3 .K643 2022 (print) | LCC R727.3 (ebook) | DDC 610.69/60952—dc23/eng/20220608
LC record available at https://lccn.loc.gov/2022016603
LC ebook record available at https://lccn.loc.gov/2022016604

British Library Cataloguing in Publication Data
A catalogue entry for this book is available from the British Library.

ISBN-13: 978-1-80041-588-1 (hbk)

Multilingual Matters
UK: St Nicholas House, 31–34 High Street, Bristol, BS1 2AW, UK.
USA: Ingram, Jackson, TN, USA.

Website: www.multilingual-matters.com
Twitter: Multi_Ling_Mat
Facebook: https://www.facebook.com/multilingualmatters
Blog: www.channelviewpublications.wordpress.com

Typeset by SAN Publishing Services.

Contents

Figures and Tables

Figures

Tables

Acknowledgments

First and foremost, I would like to express my gratitude to all the healthcare professionals, patients, their families, and local experts, who willingly volunteered their time to be involved in this project. I am especially grateful to the Japanese medical experts, Dr Daisuke Son at the Department of Community-based Family Medicine, Faculty of Medicine, Tottori University, and Dr Shinji Matsumura of Matsumura Family Clinic in Tokyo, for their professional guidance and valuable support they provided throughout my fieldwork, and to many other doctors, resident doctors, nurses and allied professionals who have inspired me.

I would like to acknowledge the academics who have helped me understand the values of concepts of patient-centredness. Dr Gabrina Pounds, in particular, has guided me for my entire time of research in applied linguistics at University of East Anglia. Her research on emotions and empathy has greatly convinced me of the importance of human sensitivity in qualitative research. Professor Andreas Musolff has also been my mentor and has given me his perspectives on healthcare discourse, always providing thoughtful and insightful opinions with great encouragement, enthusiasm and big smiles. Dr Charlotte Salter has been generous with her understanding when I struggled, and she also played a major role for me in learning the key Western consultation skills and psychosocial perspectives in the medical contexts. I will never forget all their endless guidance for the rest of my life.

I was born in a family of healthcare workers. The house I was born was located on the same premises as a medical clinic building where my uncle practiced. I grew up among medical staff and outpatients who regularly visited. I think that my family naturally demonstrated a holistic approach to caring for local patients through listening, which must have required some degree of empathy and physical and mental toughness. Special thank you and genuine respect must go to my mother, father, uncle, aunt, my partner, Luca who is a dedicated worker in social care, and all my friends. I wish to acknowledge their support and great love to complete my book and beyond.

Finally, my thanks go to Professor Jo Angouri and Professor Rebecca Piekkari, the editors of the Language at Work series, the staff at Multilingual Matters and to the reviewers for their helpful and thoughtful comments.

Acronyms

Acronym	**Referent**
FTA	Face-threatening Act
OSCE	Objective Structured Clinical Examination
PCC	Patient-centred Communication

Introduction

This book is concerned with the linguistic analysis of face-to-face clinical interactions between physicians and older adults in the context of medical consultations. This is a fieldwork-driven study, reporting empirical evidence in a previously under-researched context, in which physicians visit patients and provide in-home medical consultations with family members, in conjunction with other members of a healthcare team. All the patient–doctor exchanges reported here were collected from the professional practice in authentic settings, and the transcribed data are supplemented by one-to-one interviews with the physician participants and field notes.

Western concepts, terms such as patient/person-centred care and communication, have been disseminated worldwide and are now being embedded into real-life practice in health and social care. Previous studies investigating patient-centred communication have included a wide range of situations across the specialities, and different contexts may influence communication behaviours between patient and professionals. Existing studies on interactions between patients and healthcare providers reveal that both are important co-players in consultations and that managing this dynamic has become increasingly important to a higher quality of care of global ageing populations. The current healthcare debates involving the Covid-19 pandemic have articulated a vast range of critical reflections on effective communication in primary care, treatment and therapy, emergency care, administrative responses, and professionals' empathy and unempathic responses in the communication (Barello & Graffigna, 2020; Finset *et al.*, 2020; Holt, 2020; Houchens & Tipirneni, 2020; Musolff *et al.,* 2022). This book aims to contribute to provide: (1) a better understanding of how expressions of patients and professionals are shaped and developed, and how it could characterise the attributes of patient-centred communication; and (2) cross-cultural considerations in clinical encounters and the sociocultural differences between the UK, US, Japan and other societies in which patient-centred communication models are employed.

Regarding the terminology on patient-centred communication, while many studies use 'patient-centred care', 'person-centred care', 'people-centred care' or 'PCC' interchangeably, I use only the term 'PCC' for 'patient-centred communication' throughout this book. In addition, this differentiates between the study of patient-centred care and the study of patient-centred communication and assumes that the former includes the latter.

I.1 Scope of the Book

Chapter 1 outlines the existing conceptualisation of patient/person-centred care, with particular reference to patient-centred communication (PCC). It starts with the original concept of patient-centredness in the UK and US. The operational definition of PCC proposed by Epstein *et al.* (2005) is then discussed, followed by a review of the consultation model, Calgary-Cambridge Guide (Silverman *et al.,* 2013) and approaches to applied linguistics in healthcare settings. I then review cultural differences of the conceptualisations and applications of PCC.

Chapter 2 presents the key concepts of face and linguistic politeness and explores the discussions surrounding the classical notions of face and politeness in healthcare studies. This includes a clarification of Brown and Levinson's (1987) concepts of positive face and negative face, a discussion of social and contextual variability in linguistic behaviours, a review of the critiques of Brown and Levinson's theory and an overview of discursive approaches to politeness proposed by Locher and Watts (2005). I also take into consideration the theories of 'individualism versus collectivism' by Hofstede *et al.* ([1991] 2010) and 'high-/low-context' by Hall (1976), and the issue of cultural variability. I then turn to empirical investigations of face and politeness in medical encounters, and I suggest that Brown and Levinson's concept of face is appropriate to re-conceptualise PCC verbal dimensions for the development of the analytical categories in this study.

Chapter 3 describes the fieldwork and data and the development of the analytical framework. Since the data are based on the observational fieldwork and audio recordings of physician in-home medical consultations, I detail the methods for data collection, explaining the methodological position taken in the study, and then describe the data sample. The analysis is rooted in pragmatics and considers PCC-relevant communicative acts with reference to terminologies and definitions from the Calgary-Cambridge Guide (Silverman *et al.*, 2013) and Brown and Levinson's (1987) conceptualisations of face and politeness strategies. By drawing on both medical and linguistics concepts, the analysis advances the understanding of cultural diversity in healthcare interactions. I present a full illustration of the framework, the Face-PCC analytical categories. Short extracts from the corpus are used for illustrative purposes.

Chapter 4 explores the first PCC dimension at the beginning of the consultations, physician questioning and listening techniques in the medical consultations. This involves delivering 'Initial general remarks', 'Gradually moves from open to closed questions' and 'Repetition, paraphrasing and interpretation'. I also discuss potential non-PCC aspects (which refers to opposite examples that potentially fail to accomplish PCC), such as 'Sequence of closed questions at the beginning' and 'Interruption'. From this chapter onwards, Face-PCC elements emerging from one-to-one interviews with physician participants and longer extracts from the transcripts of the consultations are brought into the narrative interpretation of the linguistic material, to clarify some of the interpretations and further contextualise the doctors' PCC.

Chapter 5 discusses prominent features of empathy and acceptance; that is, doctors' acknowledgement of patients' concerns, fears, feelings and thoughts. I discuss the concept of clinical empathy and its background, including recent studies. Key aspects include 'Understanding and appreciation of the patient's feelings', 'Expressions of positive regard' and 'Silence as empathic anticipation'. For a potential non-PCC aspect, I discuss 'Being judgemental'.

Chapter 6 addresses physicians' attempts to understand the patient's problems and encourage shared decision-making, rather than providing one-way information. Patients' involvement was viewed as the key consultation skills in the data, suggesting that the actual use of PCC in a decision-making process can vary considerably depending on the culture. The data involved a high degree of negative politeness strategies rather than positive politeness strategies in the consultations. The key aspects include 'Sharing understanding', 'Sharing thinking' and 'Offering suggestions'. For a potential non-PCC aspect, I discuss 'No shared discussion'.

Chapter 7 concerns that physicians' responses that leave space for patients and show respect for their freedom minimise the imposition on the patient. This aspect was particularly noticeable in the in-home medical consultations: one particular cultural aspect is related to 'physical touch' and 'proximity – closeness/distance'. Key aspects involve 'Open questions that occur throughout the session', 'Checking for understanding' and 'Linguistic deference'. For potential non-PCC aspects, I discuss 'Directives' and 'Touching without asking'.

Finally, Chapter 8 deals with considerations of cultural diversity within PCC and the Western-originated model of patient/person-centredness in different cultures. It also includes difficulties encountered when conducting fieldwork, recommendations and transferring the knowledge to future professional training.

1 Introduction to Patient-centred Communication

1.1 What is Patient-centred Communication?

Supported by a growing body of health literature, descriptions of patient/person-centredness have been extensively acknowledged. According to Levenstein *et al.* (1989), the term 'patient-centred medicine' was introduced by Balint *et al.* (1970), in which a patient-centred method was described in contrast with the traditional clinical method, 'illness-centred medicine'. Discontent with the traditional 'illness-centred medicine' was well-known, as understanding the meaning of the illness *for the patient* was not aimed but only for diagnosis. Categorisations for 'disease-centred' and 'illness-centred' clinical methods were further elaborated, and Byrne and Long (1984) studied the verbal behaviours exhibited by general practitioners in consultations and developed concepts of 'doctor-centred' and 'patient-centred' behaviours. The idea of a patient-centred clinical method is closely aligned with the psychotherapeutic concept of 'client-centred therapy' proposed by Carl Rogers (Rogers, [1951] 2012, [1961] 1977).[1] There are also similarities between the patient-centred clinical method and other concepts such as person-centred and shared decision-making approaches (Stewart *et al.*, [1995] 2014).

McWhinney (1989) highlighted that, in the 1950s, Balint realised the inadequacies of the traditional clinical method for reaching a deep understanding of a patient's illness experiences and the importance of listening; Balint developed the concept of *attentive listening* and responding to a patient's '*offers*' as ways of understanding his illness (McWhinney, 1989: 31). Similarly, Levenstein *et al.* (1989) note that attentive listening allows physicians to be able to respond to the cues offered by the patient, thereby helping the patient to achieve '*the patient's agendas*'.

Levenstein *et al.* (1989: 111) described the patients' agendas and physicians' behaviours that facilitate patient-centred interviewing. Patients' agendas include expressions of (1) *ideas*, (2) *expectations*, (3) *feelings and fears* and (4) *prompts*. Patients bring their own thoughts about what is wrong with them, what might be causing it, their reasons for the visit, for which an acknowledgement or a response from the physician is anticipated. They also bring their emotional experience of the illness, which is often below the surface. The 'prompts' are signals from patients that their ideas, expectations or feelings have not yet been acknowledged or sufficiently explored; prompts can be statements that are out of context, or restatements of a problem that has already been mentioned. In turn, the physicians' behaviours include (1) *facilitative behaviours*, (2) *an acknowledgement*, (3) *cut-offs* and (4) *a return*. Facilitative behaviour refers to any verbal comments by the physician which encourages the patients' expressions of their ideas, expectations and feelings. An acknowledgement is a verbal indication that the physician has heard the patient. Conversely, cut-offs are statements in which the physician changes the subject, leaving the patient's perspective unacknowledged and blocking the patient's further expressions of their needs and views. A return occurs when a physician has cut off a patient but subsequently returns to the patient's ideas, expectations, feelings or prompts. A return is not counted as a cut-off. To achieve these two-side agendas of medical interviews, Levenstein *et al.* (1989: 119) suggest that physicians use these behaviours to integrate two perspectives, i.e. 'the medical diagnosis' and 'the patient's experience of illness' and refrain from cutting off the patient.

1.1.1 The transformation

In 1995, a comprehensive patient-centred model was developed by Stewart *et al.*, namely *Patient-Centred Medicine* (Stewart *et al.*, [1995] 2014), which is considered the most detailed and influential description on the theme (Howie *et al.*, 2004; Mead & Bower, 2000). Their recent definition suggests four components: (1) *exploring health, disease and the illness experience*; (2) *understanding the whole person*; (3) *finding common ground* and (4) *enhancing the patient–clinician relationship*. The first edition (Stewart *et al.*, 1995) comprises six components (two other components were '*incorporating prevention and health promotion*' and '*being realistic about personal limitations and issues such as the availability of time and recourses*'). Stewart *et al.* ([1995] 2014) changed the framework and explained that in the recent edition, they had incorporated the '*health promotion*' domains within '*exploring health, disease, and the illness experience*', and also, '*being realistic about personal limitations and issues such as the availability of time and recourses*' was considered not to be part of clinical care and was therefore moved to other parts.

Building on Stewart *et al.*'s earlier model of patient-centred clinical methods, Mead and Bower (2000) identify the measurable dimensions of patient-centredness through a critical review of the literature, proposing five key conceptual dimensions of patient-centredness, representing particular aspects of the patient–doctor relationship (Mead & Bower, 2000: 1088):

(1) *Biopsychosocial perspective*
(2) *The 'patient-as-person'*

(3) *Sharing power and responsibility*
(4) *The therapeutic alliance*
(5) *The 'doctor-as-person'*

These five dimensions include the principles of the four components proposed by Stewart *et al.*'s work. The first dimension, *biopsychosocial perspective,* is perceived as a key aspect that requires the physician to take a combined biological, psychological and social perspective in order to account for the wider range of problems faced by the patient. The second dimension, *'patient-as-person',* concerns understanding the patient as a person within his or her unique context since a biopsychosocial perspective alone is not sufficient for a full understanding of the patient's individual experience of illness. Third, *sharing power and responsibility* entails addressing the sociopolitical critiques of medicine – as the inevitable gap of knowledge between medical professionals and a lay patient – and requires a shift in the doctor–patient relationship from the 'co-operation-guidance' model to the 'mutual participation' model, where power and responsibility are shared with the patient. The fourth dimension, *therapeutic alliance,* refers to core therapist attitudes of empathy, congruence and unconditional positive regard and the goal of achieving a strong patient–doctor relationship. This has been endorsed by the counselling psychological approaches originally introduced by Carl Rogers (Rogers, [1951] 2012, [1961] 1977); in the counselling context, a counsellor encourages the clients to talk about themselves, using open-ended questions and showing empathy and support for the clients and their situation to establish a therapeutic alliance. The final dimension concerns the *'doctor-as-person'.* Mead and Bower (2000) note that none of the measures of patient-centredness that they reviewed covered the dimension of doctor-as-person and that this illustrates the difficulties in the operationalisation of the indicator. They conclude that, although there is agreement on types of behaviours that reflect patient-centredness (e.g. to encourage patient talk including question-asking, empathic statements, non-medical discussions and affective statements), there is little consensus on the inclusion of particular behaviours, such as doctor's information-giving towards the patient (Street, 1992).

1.1.2 Multidimensional frameworks

The conceptual ambiguity – a lack of conceptual clarity, and absence of consensus on the terminology and definition – leading to a difficulty in operationalising patient-centredness has been widely discussed (e.g. Howie *et al.*, 2004; Roter & Hall, 2004; Sharma *et al.*, 2015; Van Dulmen, 2003). For example, open-ended questions are regarded as communication behaviours that encourage patients to talk more. On the other hand, closed questions and compliance directives are generally considered as falling outside of the patient-centred domain. However, the latter is most frequently used during consultations, and some scholars identify it as fulfilling an important role, guiding the patient during the interviewing, and also as valued by the patient (Roter & Hall, 2004). Howie *et al.* (2004) note that the goal of patient-centredness is, in general, accepted as being the 'appropriate' involvement of patients in making decisions about their own care. McKinstry (2000) found that patients do not all or always want a high level of involvement in making decisions at consultations. Particularly older adults and those with more medical problems were more likely to prefer guided and doctor-led decisions, whereas younger patients and those with psychological problems tended to favour having greater participation in decision-making. McKinstry concluded that patients' expectations and their own views on management must be taken more into account (McKinstry, 2000). Similarly, Van Dulmen (2003) suggests that it can only be possible to judge the communicative effects of patient-centredness, by inquiring about each patient's individual needs and expectations.

Considering these discussions, recent studies on patient-centredness have proposed multidimensional frameworks and clearer definitions, grounded in the previous literature (Eklund *et al.*, 2019; Scholl *et al.*, 2014; Street, 2017). Scholl *et al.* (2014) conducted a systematic literature review on concept analysis and measurement scales on patient-centredness published in English or German from 1968 to 2012. Their search yielded 15 different dimensions to define the concept of patient-centredness and proposes an integrative model of patient-centredness. The 15 dimensions include: (1) essential characteristics of a clinician; (2) clinician–patient relationship; (3) clinician–patient communication; (4) patient as a unique person; (5) biopsychosocial perspective; (6) patient information; (7) patient involvement in care; (8) involvement of family and friends; (9) patient empowerment; (10) physical support; (11) emotional support; (12) integration of medical and non-medical care; (13) teamwork and teambuilding; (14) access to care and (15) coordination and continuity of care. Scholl *et al.* (2014) categorised each dimension into (a) principles of, (b) enablers of and (c) activities of patient-centred care. These dimensions are very similar to the ones identified in previous studies, but the authors note that the above describe a multitude of interrelated dimensions, rather than being independent. For example, the characteristics of the clinician influence the clinician–patient relationship; patient involvement is not possible without patient information; emotional support requires good clinician–patient communication; and communication is foundational to building a supportive relationship (Scholl *et al.*, 2014). These indicate that the integrative dimensions above promote all related patient-centred activities inductively.

On the other hand, Street (2017) focuses on differences with specific reference to the attributes of patient-centred communication (PCC), described in seven existing empirical studies, and discusses a lack of coherence in their descriptions across these studies. For example, three of the seven studies assumed PCC to be an overall clinician's communicative performance. The other four treated PCC as either an interaction process or outcome. Some measures considered PCC to be simply a ratio of how much the patient talks in relation to the doctor, whereas others assumed that PCC was manifest across multiple communication functions: information exchange, managing uncertainty, fostering relationships. Taken together with the previous conceptualisation of PCC, Street (2017: 2133) proposes a multidimensional framework for PCC which can be jointly achieved by clinicians, patients and, when appropriate, families. Street (2017) notes that the existing measures are highly clinician-centric in that they focus on the clinician's communicative performance. It can still be seen that the communicative aims above reflect clinician perspectives for the large part. It has been widely seen that PCC scales are often limited in that they assess only the clinician's communication styles, thus implicitly assuming PCC would be a clinician attribute (McCormack *et al.*, 2011).

1.1.3 Recent developments in person-centred approach

Eklund *et al.* (2019) focus on similarities and differences between two concepts: patient-centred and *person-centred* care and report that there are a number of similarities between the two concepts. The literature analysis shows that the two concepts share nine common themes: (1) empathy, (2) respect, (3) engagement, (4) relationship, (5) communication, (6) shared decision-making, (7) holistic focus, (8) individualised focus and (9) coordinated care. In addition, there are important differences regarding the goals for person-centred and patient-centred care. Person-centred care is a broader concept that includes patient-centred care, in considering 'a meaningful life for the person', whereas the goal of patient-centred care is 'a functional life for the patient' (Eklund *et al.*, 2019: 6).

Particularly in clinical settings, the concept of person-centred care has originated from the care of older adults (Eklund *et al.*, 2019), while the theory of it has often been developed in the context of dementia care and underscores the psychosocial needs of older patients. McCormack's (2003) conceptual framework for person-centred practice led to further discussion about building relationships between nurses and older adults. It posits the rights of individuals as persons as the driving force behind person-centred care and that 'it represents an attitude of respect for ordinary individuals to make rational decisions and determine their own ends' (McCormack, 2003: 202). This also means a shift away from viewing the patient as a passive target of the healthcare system towards a model in which the individual takes an active part in his or her care and decision-making (Eklund *et al.*, 2019).

As argued above, there are a number of similarities and overlaps between the two concepts: patient-centred and *person-centred* approaches.

A summary of these definitions relevant to PCC attributes above is shown in Table 1.1.

A large part of these definitions possesses complementary characteristics and leads to the mutual development of the existing approaches. The

Table 1.1 A summary of the definitions relevant to PCC in chronological order

SOURCE	DEFINITION
Levenstein *et al.* (1989)	*Patients' agendas* Patients' expressions of (1) ideas, (2) expectations, (3) feelings and fears and (4) prompts. *Physicians' behaviours* Physicians' (1) facilitative behaviours, (2) acknowledgements, (3) cut-offs and (4) returns.
Stewart *et al.* ([1995] 2014)	*Patient-Centred Medicine* comprises: 1. Exploring health, disease and the illness experience 2. Understanding the whole person 3. Finding common ground 4. Enhancing the patient–clinician relationship
Mead and Bower (2000)	The five key dimensions of patient-centredness refer to: 1. Biopsychosocial perspective 2. The 'patient-as-person' 3. Sharing power and responsibility 4. The therapeutic alliance 5. The 'doctor-as-person'
Scholl *et al.* (2014)	The 15 different dimensions that define patient-centredness are: (1) essential characteristics of a clinician; (2) clinician–patient relationship; (3) clinician–patient communication; (4) patient as a unique person; (5) biopsychosocial perspective; (6) patient information; (7) patient involvement in care; (8) involvement of family and friends; (9) patient empowerment; (10) physical support; (11) emotional support; (12) integration of medical and non-medical care; (13) teamwork and teambuilding; (14) access to care and (15) coordination and continuity of care.
Street (2017)	In a multidimensional framework, PCC: 1. Reveals the patient's perspective (beliefs, preferences, concerns, needs) 2. Explores the biopsychosocial context of the patient's health and well-being 3. Creates or reinforces trust and mutual respect in the clinician–patient relationship 4. Includes explanations of disease and treatment options in ways the patient understands 5. Has patients actively participating in the conversation and decision-making process 6. Creates shared understanding of the problem and courses of action 7. Produces decisions that are based on the evidence, consistent with patient's values, and feasible to implement.
Eklund *et al.* (2019)	The nine common themes shared between patient-centred and person-centred care: (1) empathy, (2) respect, (3) engagement, (4) relationship, (5) communication, (6) shared decision-making, (7) holistic focus, (8) individualised focus and (9) coordinated care.

next section considers the particular focus of PCC communicative domains and their definition proposed by Epstein *et al.* (2005), which is one of the most influential work in applying PCC into real-life interactions.

1.1.4 Operationalising PCC to real interactions

The work of Epstein and his colleagues has addressed a number of approaches to patient–doctor communication (Epstein, 1999, 2003; Epstein *et al.*, 1998, 2005). Specifically, Epstein has dealt with physicians' self-awareness (Epstein, 1999) and interpersonal and psychological dimensions (Epstein, 2003). Epstein *et al.* (2005: 1517) focus on patient–physician interactions and their communication domains and propose a new step in operationalising PCC. Their definition of PCC among clinicians, patient and family members includes four communication domains:

(1) Eliciting and understanding the patient's perspective – concerns, ideas, expectations, needs, feelings and functioning;
(2) Understanding the patient within his or her unique psychosocial context;
(3) Reaching a shared understanding of the problem and its treatment with the patient which is concordant with the patient's values; and
(4) Helping patients to share power and responsibility by involving them in choices to the degree that they wish.

This operational definition of PCC encompasses the previous key definitions. The first domain recognises the importance of eliciting the patient's perspective, which matches Stewart *et al.*'s ([1995] 2014) first component, 'exploring health, disease, and the illness experience' and Levenstein *et al.*'s (1989) 'Patient's agendas'. The second domain, understanding the patient's psychological and social contexts, and the third, reaching a shared understanding, correspond to Mead and Bower's (2000) 'the patient-as-person' and Stewart *et al.*'s 'understanding the whole person' and 'finding common ground'. The fourth domain, sharing power and responsibility, corresponds the domain as Mead and Bower's (2000).

Epstein *et al.* (2005) note the mediators of PCC. Patients who were trained to take a more active role in consultation (i.e. who were assigned to receive education intervention on active involvement) reported that they were more adept at eliciting information and had greater control. Those who reported changes in their health status also had an improved control of their conditions, whether or not they received the communication intervention (Williams *et al.*, 2005). The biological effect is partially mediated by changes in the patient–physician relationship, not by the increase in patient knowledge or self-care behaviours (Epstein *et al.*, 2005).

Cegala and Post (2009) examine how patients' active participation (e.g. asking questions, providing information) affects family practice physicians' use of PCC style. 'High participation' was defined as the frequency of information-seeking, information provision, assertive utterances and expressing concerns. Cegala and Post (2009) found that patients who actively participated in medical interviews influenced physicians to adopt a stronger PCC style. In particular, the physicians were more engaged in exploring the patients' disease and illness experience. However, the dimensions of understanding the whole person and establishing common ground were not significant. Physicians tended to respond by providing more information about the treatment (e.g. discussing side effects and benefits). Cegala and Post (2009) also found that highly participating patients provided considerable details about their symptoms and related medical history, and they expressed more feelings about their illness. These types of messages offered by patients were seen as having a key role in the PCC domain.

Regarding information-giving in PCC, patients with more chronic conditions are more likely to be exposed to, and responsive to, a doctor-led approach. For example, a good supply of information has a positive effect on patient satisfaction and quality of life in cancer care; however, there is significant room for improvement in the areas of emotional and psychosocial support to patients (McCormack *et al.*, 2011; Ouwens *et al.*, 2010). Epstein and Street (2007) suggest that PCC (as defined in Epstein *et al.*, 2005) may be particularly effective in cancer care, and they go on to give examples of patient-centred clinician behaviours, including the provision of sufficient information and clear, jargon-free explanations. They also argue that it is essential for clinicians to discover the way in which cancer patients want to be involved in decision-making and make appropriate adaptations and that:

> Conversely, clinicians who have limited perceptiveness or a fixed communication style will have less adaptability and will find they interact with some patients effectively but have considerable difficulty with others. (Epstein & Street, 2007: 8)

Taylor (2009) also gave a warning about styles of information-giving, claiming that patient-centredness is less likely to be valued by some patients in general practice and by older patients who may be more comfortable with paternalism. The author points out that clinicians require specific skills to recognise the preferred style of the patient with more medical conditions – how much they want to participate – and to adapt sufficiently to respond accordingly.

In sum, the studies reviewed above have determined the properties that characterise patient-centredness and PCC. While the majority of them seem to take a comparatively critical view on the conceptual ambiguity, there are also studies that further develop and demonstrate components of PCC by drawing on the commonalities. The next section will take a closer look at communication process skills in the PCC domain in the context of medical education.

1.1.5 Calgary-Cambridge Guide

Regarding teaching, assessing and researching PCC, the Calgary-Cambridge Guide proposed by Silverman *et al.* (2013) is regarded as a comprehensive framework of skills for doctor–patient communication. The guide is developed to address health professionals' and educators' needs and for teaching core clinical skills in medical education and post-graduate training and is widely used in medical schools in the UK, Europe and North America (Brown *et al.*, 2016). The guide's basic framework is designed to correspond to a structured process of medical consultations, which consists of the following core tasks: 'Initiating the session'; 'Gathering information'; 'Physical examinations'; 'Explanation and planning' and 'Closing the session'. In addition to these tasks, there are two continuous threads throughout the consultation: 'Building the relationship' and 'Providing structure' (see Figure 1.1).

The framework is subdivided into 73 communication process skills, and each item is further elaborated. For example, specific process skills for 'Gathering information' are designed to explore the patient's problems by seeking both biomedical and patient perspectives. Statements made by patients regarding family, beliefs, work demands, struggles and life crisis that contextualise illness are regarded as pertaining to the psychosocial context. For the doctor's communication process of 'Gathering information', 11 process skills are illustrated. Of these skills, 'Questioning techniques' are particularly elaborated and warned. The guide defines 'open (divergent) questions' as questions for which the doctor introduces an area of enquiry without unduly shaping or focusing the content of the response. 'Closed (convergent) questions', in contrast, are questions for which a

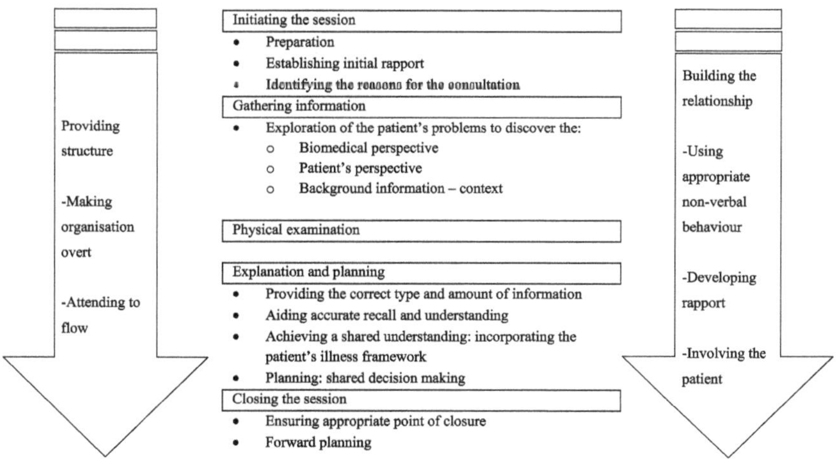

Figure 1.1 The Calgary-Cambridge Guide framework (Silverman *et al.*, 2013: 19)
Reproduced with the permission of the licensor.

specific and one-word answer such as yes or no is usually expected from the patient (Silverman *et al.*, 2013: 74):

- open – *'Tell me about your headaches'*
- more directive but still open – *'What makes your headaches better or worse?'*
- closed – *'Do you ever wake up with a headache in the morning?'*

The guide emphasises that both open and closed questions are essential but have different ends. Silverman *et al.* (2013: 75) introduce the 'open-to-closed-cone' (found by Goldberg *et al.*, 1983, in Silverman *et al.*, 2013: 78), which starts with open questions and later gradually moves to closed questions. This technique first obtains a picture of the problem in the patients' words, and moves towards specific aspects of the problem, still using open questions. Closed questions may eventually be used to elicit finer details that the patient may have omitted. The ratio of open to closed questions has been significantly correlated with the patient's talkativeness and contributions. This is in accordance with early studies of PCC, showing that that the use of open questions greatly encourages the patient to tell their story and is particularly important at the beginning of the consultation.

The task 'Explanation and planning' is designed to provide explanations that relate the patients' problems and their understanding of these problems and to involve the patient by planning the treatment collaboratively. This task particularly addresses the doctor's use of language, which patients often do not understand and that also may have an impact on the patient's involvement in the interview. For the process skills of 'Explanation and planning', 35 process skills are provided (e.g. 'gives information in chunks and checks for understanding', 'provides opportunities and encourages patient to contribute', etc.). These skills concern providing the correct amount of information, aiding accurate recall, and achieving a shared understanding. In the PCC domain, these characteristics are considered particularly helpful in enabling patients to share power and responsibility by involving them.

Communicating with older patients is addressed by the guide. Special consideration is given to listening to impaired or partially sighted people. Doctors need to use the skills of triadic interviewing with patients who are accompanied by a family member or friend. Key communication dimensions with older patients include asking clarifying questions, time-framing, summarising, picking up cues, checking out, using clear language, and also supporting mutual discussion of resources and responsibility, discussion of relevant aspects of the patient's life context, and showing a caring attitude from the physician and continuity of care (Silverman *et al.*, 2013: 242). Although some of the communication dimensions can be age-related issues, all the skills are nonetheless important elements of PCC.

1.1.6 Overview of approaches to applied linguistics in healthcare settings

There has been a vast volume of work on discourse-based linguistic studies in healthcare settings over the past three decades (e.g. Atkins *et al.*, 2016; Holmes & Stubbe, 2015; Locher, 2017; Locher & Schnurr, 2017; Ordóñez-López & Edo-Marzá, 2016; Roberts & Sarangi, 2003, 2005; Rudolf von Rohr *et al.*, 2019; Sarangi, 2005, 2010a, 2010b; Sarangi & Roberts, 1999). The publication *Talk, Work and Institutional Order: Discourse in Medical, Mediation and Management Settings* by Sarangi and Roberts (1999) offers theoretical insights and methodological tools for discourse analytic and pragmatic studies in health and social care. The authors shed new light on an interdisciplinary approach to professional discourse in a wide range of institutional settings, with the focus on 'how professional knowledge and identities are constituted in interaction within an over-arching institutional order' (Sarangi & Roberts, 1999: 43). Discourse analysis combines the content of each turn of talk, how verbal interactions are sequenced and managed, and the speakers' choices of vocabulary, grammar, rhetoric and communicative situations. The majority of this applied linguists' work takes an interdisciplinary approach to individual–professional or interprofessional talk from an 'outsider' view. The outsiders can bridge the gap between academic research and its practical relevance within many other professional settings by identifying problems and offering solutions (Roberts & Sarangi, 2003, 2005; Sarangi, 2005).

In relation to PCC, applied linguists have offered perspectives as experts of communicative domains. For example, Roberts *et al.* (2004) point out that patient-centred models strongly encourage doctors to let their patients talk; however, they hardly recognise the fact that there could be problems with patients' abilities to produce coherent, intelligible narratives (2004: 160). To a certain extent, models of medical consultations assume that the patient can describe symptoms and that doctors can elicit information without difficulty. The issue of how discourse strategies are managed in real life settings of professional communication has been tackled within politeness research that focuses on power dynamics (Holmes & Stubbe, 2015; Locher, 2017; Locher & Schnurr, 2017). Most of this research is data-driven and draws on qualitative sociolinguistic methodologies, such as discourse analysis and conversation analysis. Holmes and Stubbe's (2015) publication, *Power and Politeness in the Workplace: A Sociolinguistic Analysis of Talk at Work,* presents a number of authentic discourse contexts, demonstrating how much analysts can discover from close readings of data, and elaborating important dimensions in which participants negotiate and resolve miscommunication and problematic issues (2015: 163). Miscommunication that occurs with linguistic and ethnic minorities in medical encounters is also a well-researched area (Hilder *et al.*, 2019; Moss & Roberts, 2005; Roberts, 2009; Roberts & Moss, 2003).

Another critique relevant to communication skills training is Atkins *et al.*'s (2016) sociolinguistic analysis of talk in Objective Structured Clinical Examination (OSCE) interactions. The OSCE is used in countries worldwide to assess clinical competence for undergraduates and postgraduates in medical education. Simulated patients are lay people or professional actors trained to act as a patient with a particular condition in the OSCE; the nature of the role-play with simulated patients is considered as an 'artificial context'. Atkins *et al.* (2016) examined how far simulated consultations reflect real-life clinical encounters. They found that simulation consultations undoubtedly have a place in formative learning but may distort assessment of professional communication. These findings support ongoing critiques of simulations – what is being assessed is not real communication but the ability to voice a credible appearance of such communication. This has much to do with the 'image' that the speaker projects of him or herself towards the listener (which is more fully discussed in the next chapter).

1.2 Cultural Differences in Patient–Doctor Relationship

Traditionally, the patient–physician relationship in Japan was strongly hierarchical and paternalistic, very similar to the old relationship in which Western general practitioners used to have little regard for the patient's opinions and where questions from the patient were considered as a lack of recognition of the doctor's abilities (McKinstry, 1992). Yajima and Takayanagi (1998) delineated the Japanese traditional styles in clinical communication, similarly, explaining that Japanese patients tended to hesitate when posing questions to doctors because such behaviour can be perceived as a challenge to the doctor's professionalism and can risk disrupting their relationship. Early cultural studies also revealed that traditionally a relatively low value is placed on verbalisation in Japanese society; instead, more particular emphasis is placed on non-verbal factors such as facial expressions and tone of voice (Hirota, 1992; Maynard, 1993; Takayama *et al.*, 2001).

The issue of patients' perceptions about physicians' information-giving and guidance is addressed by Hirota (1992) and Uchida *et al.* (1999). Hirota (1992) conducted interviews with patients visiting hospital outpatient services and found that most patients felt hesitant about asking questions or requesting explanation about their prescriptions, because the patients did not want to offend or disturb their physicians. Subsequently, a questionnaire survey was conducted in the same hospital which reported that 76% of patients wished to gain more information from their physicians and about 20% preferred more doctor-led styles. The latter respondents were mostly older patients. Hirota concluded that in hospital settings, the stage had not been reached yet where doctors provided a good supply of information that met the patients' expectations.

While the Western concept of PCC assumes that the patient is a modern individual who makes rational judgements and decisions, the preference for doctor-led styles could still be rooted in Japan. Ishikawa *et al.* (2002) claimed that Japanese physicians significantly focused on biomedical topics; compared to two previous studies conducted in the UK and the Netherlands, the proportion of statements showing concerns and reassurance was smaller in their data. Ishikawa *et al.* (2002) also observed that Japanese consultations included a higher proportion of social behaviours such as laughter. Another comparative study between the US and Japanese medical consultations showed that Japanese patient–doctor interactions included more silence (30% for the total time of consultation) than those in the US (8.2%); in contrast, the ratios of total speech between them were almost similar (Ohtaki *et al.*, 2003).

Ishikawa and Yamazaki (2005) discussed the adoption of Western concepts of patient–physician relationship from the perspective of socio-cultural factors. The authors examined the extent to which Western-based mutual participation models of the relationship can be compatible with Japanese society, based on a comparative analysis between Japanese and Western cultures. Two key factors play a role with regard to the uptake of the Western model in Japan: 'family' and 'communication styles'. Placing a higher value on collectivistic behaviours rather than on individuals may be in conflict with the new principle of patient participation. Assuming the autonomy of individuals may, therefore, not be appropriate when addressing healthcare issues in Japanese contexts. Since the interactional styles may differ (Ishikawa *et al.*, 2002; Ohtaki *et al.*, 2003), patient–physician relationship in the Japanese context should be considered within the context of a triadic relationship of patient, family and physician.

Matusitz and Spear (2015) compared the communication styles between patients and doctors in three Asian countries – Pakistan, Japan and Thailand – with those in the US. Their findings showed that the patient–doctor relationship in the Asian countries tended to be more hierarchical and paternalistic compared to that of the US, and family members were more highly involved in the patient's decision-making. Matusitz and Spear (2015) concluded that the US-style doctor–patient communication model is not very applicable in the three Asian countries, including Japan. The authors provide explanations by drawing on the traditional collectivistic perspectives and cultural comparisons, based on the religious or philosophical dimension of the healthcare background. However, there still seems to be a lack of investigation into why the adoption of the US model is problematic and what sort of elements in the patient–doctor communication models are practical or impractical, with particular reference to the pressure imposed on the system by an ageing society.

The differences in social values between the UK and Japan have often been the subject of cross-cultural comparison from anthropological perspectives, such as individualism versus collectivism, femininity versus masculinity, and Christianity versus Confucianism (Hall, 1976; Hofstede, 1984, 1991; Liu *et al.*, 2011). These social perspectives highlight the importance of the relationship between the communicative aspects and cultural variations in care contexts. However, to date, few studies have specifically focused on the cultural variations of the Western models of clinical communication. Investigating the characteristics of verbal behavioural elements – identifying the PCC verbal elements – is very important in developing the interpersonal skills of physicians.

1.2.1 Importing the theories into Japan

Patient–doctor communication began to be further addressed after 2000, and the importance of teaching the Western originated patient-centred concept has been emphasised by medical educators (e.g. Koizumi, 2010; Matsumura & Minowa, 2007; Miyata & Mukohara, 2015; Okutani *et al.*, 2007). This trend is being further accelerated with the introduction of the OSCE in medical education.

In one of the commonly used textbooks on medical interviews (a summary of the educational materials used in Japanese medical school is presented in Appendix 9.2), Saito (2000: 53) introduces five communication skills that reinforce the building of patient–doctor relationships and addressing patients' emotions. These skills are adapted from *The Medical Interview* proposed by Cole in the US (Cole & Bird, 1994).

(1) Reflection (e.g. *'You seem to be frustrated'*)
(2) Legitimation (e.g. *'It is a painful situation, as anyone can see'*)
(3) Support (e.g. *'I would like to do as much as I can'*)
(4) Partnership (e.g. *'Let's think about this problem together'*)
(5) Respect (e.g. *'While in a painful situation, you have been working hard'*) (Saito, 2000: 53)

Saito regards these five skills as doctors' empathic communication and notes that empathy can be achieved through listening techniques such as using nods, repeating and paraphrasing to clarify what a patient is saying, and in particular, avoiding expressing sympathy which may expose a patient to emotional stress (Saito, 2000: 52).

Such an association between empathy and listening techniques is recognised in the Japanese version of the OSCE assessment guidelines, which have been compiled by a non-profit organisation, Common Achievement Tests Organization (2020). Medical students are advised that performing empathic communication skills will help them to achieve patient-centred consultations and that they will be assessed on their listening attitudes, which are the particular focus of these educational instructions. The assessment checklist for medical interview skills includes six main sections: (1) opening; (2) empathic communication; (3) gathering information–medical history; (4) gathering information–psychological and social background; (5) providing information; (6) closing session. Each section is then subdivided into further skills. For example, the checklist for empathic communication can be summarised as follows (Common Achievement Tests Organization, 2020: 19):

- Maintain eye contact with the patient, not only when asking questions but also when listening to the patient;
- Take an appropriate posture when listening to the patient;
- Take an attentive listening stance by using open-ended questions throughout the consultation;
- Use fillers and nods to facilitate communication with the patient;
- Use appropriate listening techniques, for example, avoid interrupting the patient;
- Use appropriate verbal techniques (e.g. volume, tone of voice, paraphrasing, repeating, summarising and/or confirming the patient's statements) and
- Express empathy towards the patient's feelings and circumstances verbally and non-verbally; i.e. only using verbal expressions is not enough.

As these examples show, non-verbal signs of listening are specified. In this regard, Maynard (1993) previously described that Japanese speakers used nods and fillers three times more frequently compared to American English speakers. Indeed, Kita and Ide (2009) note that in Japanese conversations, these behaviours may even be displayed by the turn-holder and not just by the listener; nods tend to elicit further nods from the conversational partner. In clinical settings, Saito (2000: 47) defines listening as attitudes that help the patients express themselves and make the patients feel accepted; showing curiosity non-verbally is seen as conveying a positive message and brings therapeutic effects. More specific characteristics include silence, encouragements and echoing. Although the importance of active listening has been most frequently mentioned by scholars in health research, it is more significant in combination with cultural behavioural aspects such as nods and postures.

The Calgary-Cambridge Guide (Silverman *et al.*, 2013) has been adapted to a Japanese textbook written by Mukohara (2006) for both undergraduate and postgraduate levels. Mukohara introduces a framework of physician communication competence based on two different Western models: the Calgary-Cambridge Guide (Silverman *et al.*, 2013) and a US-originated clinical communication skills model, the Macy Model of Doctor–Patient Communication (Kalet *et al.*, 2004). The latter model highlights three main functions: (1) gathering data, (2) establishing a therapeutic rapport and (3) educating the patient. These three areas organise a number of skills into a series of different tasks that structure the flow of the interview. Mukohara's basic framework is identical to the Calgary-Cambridge Guide: a set of diagrams outlines five phases ('initiating the session', 'gathering information', 'physical examination', 'explanation and planning' and 'closing the session') with two continuous threads throughout the tasks ('building the relationship' and 'providing structure'). Mukohara (2006) applies 27 behavioural items from the Macy Model into his framework. Specific reasons for why this modification was taken are not given; however, he lists three reasons why these two Western models are useful in Japanese settings:

(1) These Western models are premised on wider-scale research evidence that validates the importance of communication skills;
(2) The models address specific attitudes and issues (such as the patient's anger, addictions). This helps doctors to identify which skills they should concentrate on in each task. The Western models focus on task objectives that are likely to pertain to wider clinical settings;
(3) The models are well-balanced in terms of the concept. The traditional model of taking the patient's medical history in the early period had a strong emphasis on gathering information without conducting physical examinations and educating patients; the Western models balance all these aspects. (Mukohara, 2006: 4)

Mukohara also briefly introduces the work of Epstein on physician self-awareness (Epstein, 1999) that underlies the conceptual idea of PCC. These indicate that the PCC concept is certainly acknowledged among Japanese educators and encouraged to be taught in Japanese medical education settings.

1.2.2 Unclear definitions of patient-centredness

One commonly recognised problem in those textbooks is that the definition of patient-centredness remains unclear, while the term is overused (Maeda, 2005: 12). There are descriptions of how the traditional style of relationships impedes the development of communication skills. Fujisaki *et al.* (2015) explain that there is a misunderstanding about perceptions of doctors' communication styles, which are often interpreted as doctors' styles of hearing and retrieving information for diagnosis; this misunderstanding has inhibited medical education (Fujisaki *et al.*, 2015: 182). Matsushige (2010) provides a critique of the conceptualisation and the barriers to it from a sociological perspective summarised as follows: (1) there is no definition of the term commonly shared in Japan, (2) there is a lack of clarity regarding what is to be done by health professionals to realise patient-centredness; (3) it is unclear what the patient him/herself needs to do to realise patient-centred interaction; (4) it is unclear how the knowledge of medical expertise and the concept of patient-centredness can be integrated (Matsushige, 2010: 2).

Although efforts have been made to promote a patient-centred approach among professionals at both organisational and institutional levels, discussions that draw on shared perceptions of the public remain inconclusive. The definition and implementation of PCC are directed to more institution-led styles in a broad range of healthcare fields. In an oncology setting, Takayama *et al.*'s (2001) study confirms that a patient-centred and facilitative style was significantly related to lower anxiety levels (Takayama *et al.*, 2001). The study found that cancer patients evaluated their physician's communication according to the extent to which they were 'accepting', 'patient-centred', 'attentive' and 'facilitative'. The results showed that when the physician's communication style was evaluated highly, patients' post-consultation anxiety remained low, even among those patients with unfavourable examination results. Takayama *et al.* (2001: 1336) note that, traditionally, a relatively low value is placed on verbalisation in Japanese society; instead, more particular emphasis is placed on non-verbal factors such as facial expressions and tone of voice. The physicians' 'accepting' attitudes received the highest score by the patients, followed by 'patient-centred' and 'facilitative' attitudes, which were well in accordance with the patients' lower anxiety levels. This means that a physician's attitude along with 'less verbalisation' were valued by the patients in the cancer setting.

Kisa *et al.* (2011) studied physicians' outpatient consultations in a rural region with a high population of older patients, using questionnaires for both patients and physicians to elicit their views on the physicians' patient-centred approach. Their findings show that patient satisfaction was much higher than physician satisfaction. Both patients and physicians were satisfied with their first encounters; however, the level of satisfaction varied for specific categories: 98.4% of patients but only 62.3% of physicians were satisfied with the 'emotional support' they received/offered; and 91.8% of patients but only 68.9% of physicians were satisfied with the 'interaction in general'. The patients felt satisfied regardless of the physician's opinion, and patient satisfaction was not completely associated with physician satisfaction. These results in the traditional setting would also indicate that the patients might prefer professional-led styles, resulting in higher satisfaction with physicians' guidance.

Kuga *et al.* (2016) report that the practice of shared decision-making, which is an important factor in patient-centred medicine in primary care, is not prevalent in Japan. They conducted a survey for physicians in Tokyo where they evaluated the decision-making methods for treatment using a five-point scale: 'paternalism', 'close-to-paternalism', 'informed consent', 'shared decision-making' and 'informed decision-making'. The most frequently used method was 'informed consent' at 40.8%, for which the doctor selects a suitable option, provides explanations and selects it after gaining the patient's agreement. This was closely followed by 'close-to-paternalism' at 38%, 'shared decision-making' at 14.6% and 'paternalism'

6.4%. Most of the doctors were in their 50s and had gained their experience in hospital environments. Kuga *et al.* (2016) explain that younger doctors tended to opt for informed consent, while experienced doctors preferred paternalism.

Recent studies have investigated the attitudes of medical students and residents to patient-centred care. The next section briefly shows Japanese medical students' perception of PCC measures and their lack of confidence.

1.2.3 Medical students' perceptions

In order to explore medical students' receptivity to patient-centred attitudes, Ishikawa *et al.* (2014) investigated their confidence in performing medical interviews. First-year resident physicians at a hospital in Tokyo were asked about their confidence. The authors found that the residents had high confidence in their skills to gather information and build relationships with patients; however, they felt least confident in the tasks of sharing information and planning treatment. The authors explain that undergraduate medical education tends to concentrate on teaching students how to gather information from the patient in the setting of a first-visit outpatient consultation and that explanation and negotiation skills tend to be neglected. In addition, communication skills training in postgraduate education has not been as well established as in undergraduate programmes; instead, residents are expected to learn from their everyday interactions with patients (Ishikawa *et al.*, 2014).

According to their most recent study of first-year medical students' residency programme, a significant decline in patient-centred attitudes was observed (Ishikawa *et al.*, 2018). The educational focus on gathering information and students' performances correlated as strongly as in their previous study (Ishikawa *et al.*, 2014: 364). Circumstances in clinical training (e.g. heavy workloads and tight schedules) are considered as one of the possible reasons for the decline in their attitudes towards sharing information.

There seems to be persistent confusion about the concept of patient-centredness, and PCC tends to be associated with listening and gathering information phases, which indicates that more difficulties are found in developing the skills required for shared decision-making. Lack of confidence in utilising shared decision-making has also been seen among first-year residents in English-speaking countries (e.g. Caldwell, 2008; Legare & Witteman, 2013).

1.3 Summary

Although scholars and educators discuss the concepts differently, most descriptions published in the UK and US share the key elements of PCC or are in some sense complementary. In the publications in Japan, there are little concrete definitions of PCC, while the work of Epstein has been briefly introduced in one of the educational textbooks (Mukohara, 2006). I conclude that Epstein *et al.*'s operational definitions of PCC (2005) are appropriate for this interactional linguistic analysis, allowing me to focus on verbal dimensions and interactions in medical consultations between older patients and physicians. Furthermore, the Calgary-Cambridge Guide (Silverman *et al.*, 2013) provides the foundation for the exploration of physicians' communicative behaviours in the analysis of this study because the skills' categories have applications internationally. Based on these definitions of PCC above, these communicative aspects are revisited in the next chapter from the pragmatic notion of face and linguistic politeness. In particular, I review the extent to which politeness concepts have been applied in this study, with particular reference to cultural differences.

1.4 Objectives and Research Questions

The specific objective of this study is to assess the adoption of the concepts and theories of PCC in real-life interactions between older patients and physicians. In particular, it aims to clarify which elements of the concept and theories of PCC are practical and could, therefore, be successfully adopted and how that might be best achieved. Ultimately, it is hoped that the findings in this book can be utilised to develop effective communication skills training for healthcare professionals, geriatricians, medical students and trainees, and social workers, to improve the quality of elderly care. The aims of the study are met by the following specific objectives:

(1) Identify potential barriers to incorporating the concept and model of PCC.
(2) Observe communication practice in medical consultations in the care context for older patients and elicit physicians' views of communication skills.
(3) Consider the implications of the findings from the above and produce a set of recommendations aimed at medical educators and physicians and students.

In order to achieve these main objectives, the following four Research Questions are addressed:

(1) To what extent are principles and practice of the patient–doctor relationship in Japan drawn from the Western approach to medical consultations; more specifically:
    (a) How is this demonstrated in the experience of Japanese physicians and older patients?

(b) How is this demonstrated in actual consultation practice with older patients?

(2) What are the implications of the above for medical educators and future doctors?

Note

(1) The concept of client-centred therapy is a non-directive therapy, suggesting that the therapist should not direct the client, should not be judgemental on the client's feelings and should not offer suggestions or solutions. The first publication of *Client-Centred Therapy: Its Current Practice, Implications, and Theory* (Rogers, 1951) created a major influence in helping professions (Kirschenbaum & Jourdan, 2005). At first, Rogers used the term 'non-directive therapy', 'client-centred', then 'person-centred' to describe his approach to counselling and psychotherapy.

2 Face and Linguistic Politeness

This chapter continues exploring interpersonal concerns that arise in medical consultation contexts. Chapter 1 introduced the concept and definitions of patient/person-centredness and zoomed in on the critiques and discussions raising in different cultures. Chapter 2 focuses on the pragmatic notion of 'face' and 'linguistic politeness' theories. Face and politeness theory has been widely applied to empirical investigations in encounters in health and social care settings, in which politeness has been studied with reference to the power dynamics, social beliefs and structure of patient-professional consultations (Locher & Schnurr, 2017; Mullany, 2009). This has included a wide range of health settings, such as hospital wards, telephone consultations and electronic communication via emails and elderly care facilities (e.g. Backhaus, 2017; Grainger, 2004; Lambert, 1996; Makoni & Grainger, 2002; Norris & Rowsell, 2003). Empirical evidence from these studies has provided useful resources to inform communication training for professionals and has raised awareness of the importance of the language that they use towards patients. *The Journal of Politeness Research* has also encouraged the application of politeness theory to health-related research, publishing the special issues 'Politeness in health care settings' (Mullany, 2009; Van Der Bom & Grainger, 2015).

Since its publication in 1987, *Politeness: Some universals in language usage* by Brown and Levinson has exercised widespread influence not only in arts and humanities but also in behavioural sciences such as cognitive psychology, adding to the understanding of social cognitive phenomena (Holtgraves, 2005). The classical work of Brown and Levinson's model has remained influential in health professional education because of the clear utility. The Brown and Levinson's theory assumes that linguistic politeness could be seen as a universal phenomenon, and its framework includes 40 linguistic strategies used by an 'actor' (a social member who is a fluent speaker of a language). However, this theory has drawn criticisms from numerous researchers, particularly from East Asian scholars, in terms of its theoretical construct, conceptualisation of face and variability in other languages. These critiques have led to further discussions on the issues and produced a large number of research evidence, contributing to further developments of politeness theory. One of the key publications, Locher and Watts (2005), focuses on the conceptualisation of 'relational work'. Their claim provides an updated theory of politeness, proposing that politeness is a discursive concept and must be seen in relation to other types of interpersonal meaning. However, in a shift to the discursive approach to politeness, further debates have arisen, and the 'utility' of the notion of politeness has been questioned and re-examined (Haugh, 2007).

This chapter presents the key concepts and features of face and linguistic politeness and explore the social and contextual variability in the relevant linguistic behaviours. The main critiques of the politeness theory in the early 1990s and the important debates surrounding 'the discursive approach to politeness' are discussed. I review contextual considerations, dealing with the concept of 'individualism versus collectivism' (Hofstede *et al.*, [1991] 2010) and components of cultural variability, as well as briefly addressing key aspects of Japanese linguistic politeness. I then discuss empirical investigations of linguistic politeness, providing summaries of the main criticisms of Brown and Levinson's (1987) politeness theory, especially those by East Asian researchers. This chapter concludes that, in spite of its limitations, the classical work of Brown and Levinson's politeness theory has provided an efficient and workable tool for conceptualising the patient's face.

2.1 What is Brown and Levinson's Politeness Theory?

The central concept of Brown and Levinson's (1987) politeness theory is based on the notion of 'face' and 'face-work', which was introduced by Goffman's essay, *Interaction Ritual* (1967). Goffman (1967) defined 'face' as describing an image of oneself delineated in terms of approved social attributes – an image that others may share. Brown and Levinson referred to it as 'the public self-image that every member [of a society] wants to claim for himself' (1987: 61). They assumed that most conversations could include 'face-threatening acts (FTAs)' to either the hearer or speaker. Politeness is described as strategies that attempt to mitigate the threat of FTA. Thus, professional practice in a social context would be directed by the speaker's desire to convey their own positive image as well as to mitigate the potential of face threats to others.

Brown and Levinson first presupposed that a 'Model Person' (MP) has two special traits: 'rationality' and 'face' (1987: 58). Regarding face, Brown and Levinson identified two aspects – or double traits, reflecting two sides of the concept – 'negative face' and 'positive face'. The former refers to the speakers' desire to be independent, be unimpeded and self-autonomous; the latter is the want to be accepted, praised and appreciated for an affirmative self-image (1987: 62). Regarding 'rationality', Brown and Levinson claimed that members of a society 'act' rationally to achieve a communicative goal and that the rational behaviours contain the ability to choose means that most satisfy the goal (1987: 65). In addition, they formed a hypothesis that certain kinds of interactive acts intrinsically threaten the participant's face, such as orders, requests, suggestions, advice, offers, compliments and expressions of envy or admiration (1987: 66).

For example, making a request may threaten the hearer's negative face (that is the want to be unimpeded), as it makes demands on his or her time and effort to achieve the request, rather than the hearer's positive face (which is the want to be appreciated). The speaker may, more or less consciously, try to minimise threatening face by selecting the most suitable strategy, such as being indirect when requesting (e.g. the use of question and hedge as in *Can (Could) you pass the salt?*, the use of sentences including insertion of please such as in *Can you please shut the door?* or the use of phrases from which requests may be implied in context, even though not literally stated, such as *I need some glue* or *I am looking for some glue*). In other cases, the act is performed 'baldly', which involves the most direct, clear and unambiguous ways (e.g. the request is made explicitly, as in *Shut the door!*).

On the other hand, most everyday linguistic behaviours between intimates, such as sharing interests and approval, are oriented to the hearer's positive face (1987: 101). Unlike negative politeness, positive politeness may not necessarily be redressive of a particular face-want infringed by FTA. Negative politeness redresses the imposition itself made by the speaker, whereas positive politeness covers more general acceptance towards the hearer's own wants (1987: 101). The speaker may take notice of the hearer's condition or noticeable changes (e.g. attentiveness to the hearer as in *You must be hungry, it's a long time since breakfast. How about some lunch?*) or approve of hearers' remarkable possessions or qualities with 'exaggerated' approval and/or lexical or grammatical intensification (e.g. the use of intensifying modifiers as in *What a fantastic garden you have!*). Brown and Levinson (1987) noted that only 'exaggeration' can be a feature that distinguishes redressive positive politeness from normal everyday intimate language. They argue that exaggerated expression offers a marker of the face-redress aspect of positive politeness, which can sincerely express 'I want your positive face to be satisfied', even if the speaker cannot behave with total sincerity (1987: 101). The insincerity of exaggerated language behaviour is compensated by the implication that the speaker sincerely wants the hearer's positive face to be enhanced. This will be further reviewed and discussed in Section 2.4 *Empirical work in medical encounters* with regard to the use of praise expressions by healthcare providers towards their patients.

In summary, the speaker has five main possible strategies to do, or avoid, or minimise FTA (see Figure 2.1): (1) do the act without redressive action, baldly (as illustrated above); (2) positive politeness (redress acts

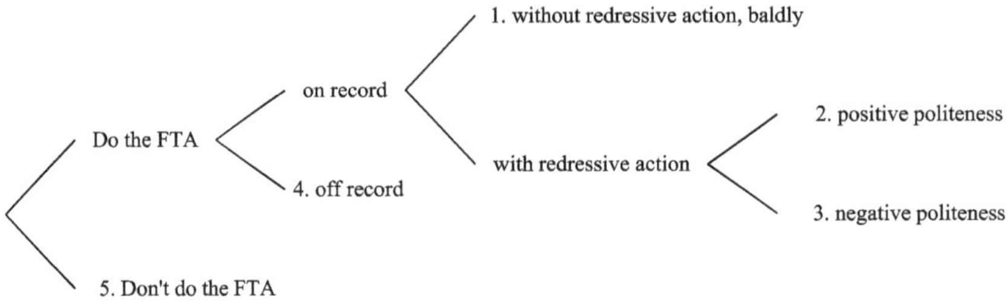

Figure 2.1 Possible strategies for doing FTAs (Brown & Levinson, 1987: 69)
Reproduced with the permission of the licensor.

directed to the hearer's positive face as illustrated above); (3) negative politeness (as in the indirect forms illustrated above); (4) 'off record' as an act that is done in a way that is not possible to attribute a clear communicative intention to it; the speaker leaves it up to the hearer to decide how the act is to be intended. Examples would include the interpretation of expressions such as *I am tired. A cup of tea would help* where the implied request may be acknowledged or ignored; (5) don't do the FTA.

The strategies on record and off record can be distinguished by whether the speaker's intention is clear to the hearer (when going on record) or whether there is more than one attributable intention so that the speaker cannot be held to have committed himself to one particular intent (Brown & Levinson, 1987: 69). The range of positive and negative politeness consists of 40 main strategies, and these are illustrated as interaction strategies oriented to speakers' and hearers' perspectives in communication. 'Positive politeness strategies' are approach-based and aimed towards the hearers' positive face, whereas 'negative politeness strategies' are essentially avoidance-based and directed to redressing hearers' negative face (1987: 70). The selection of the most suitable FTA strategies depends on the social distance (D) between speaker and hearer, the relative power (P) between them and the absolute ranking (R) of impositions in the particular culture (1987: 74). In addition, using jokes and in-group language and presenting familiarity as 'you are the same as me' is considered a positive politeness strategy. On the other hand, negative politeness strategies also focus on effacing the speaker themselves, and maintaining formality and restraint, such as being indirect, using hedges and giving deference.

This politeness model assumes that the use of verbal strategies in social interactions can be observed across cultures, which suggests that 'the mutual knowledge of members' public self-image or face, and the social necessity to orient oneself to it in interaction, are universal' (1987: 62). However, this claim, the universalism of the distinction, has given rise to debates over cultural variation. Particularly, a number of scholars studying non-Western languages have re-considered the notion of face and politeness with regard to those languages. The main criticism from the perspective of East Asian languages and discussions of a move to 'discursive approaches to politeness' will be reviewed in the following section.

2.2 Criticisms of Brown and Levinson's Theory

2.2.1 Claims from East Asian scholars

In the early 1990s, the face and politeness theory was the subject of discussions among East Asian linguists (Gu, 1990; Ide, 1989; Ide *et al.*, 1992; Mao, 1994; Matsumoto, 1988). Matsumoto (1988: 404) argued that the concept of 'negative face', as the want to be unimpeded, would be an alien notion to Japanese culture. She explained that, in general, Japanese speakers prioritise the maintenance and acknowledgement of social relations with other members (of a social group) over their personal goals, which dominates any interactions, rather than defending their individual territories (1988: 408). For example, an expression used as a common courtesy in Japan is '*Douzo yoroshiku onegaishimasu* (Please consider me favourably)'. This phrase is used in various situations, such as when introducing oneself to someone, or closing a meeting, or expressing a hope to have a good outcome or relationship with the other person. In Brown and Levinson's framework, this expression '*Please consider...*' can be projected as an imposition on the hearer's freedom of action and classified as a 'request', which may be threatening the hearer's negative face. However, the expression is not considered as a request in Japan. Instead, it is associated with enhancing the hearer's self-image, because this indicates that the hearer has the ability to attend to the speaker's desire, and the action of stating the expression is socially expected and appreciated as essential for relationship-building. This also implies that the hearer is regarded as holding a higher position in the context, and the hearer's positive face must be satisfied by being acknowledged in the expression. Thus, this should be seen as a positive politeness strategy that attends to the hearer's positive face (Matsumoto, 1988: 410).

Matsumoto also claimed that polite forms called 'honorifics', which are lexical and morphological encodings in the Japanese grammatical system, cannot be considered as forms of negative politeness strategy to defuse potential FTA, as proposed in Brown and Levinson's theory. Brown and Levinson (1987: 277) were aware of the origin and system of the Japanese honorifics and referred to them as face-preserving strategies. However, Matsumoto (1988) explained that the use of honorifics is not a negative politeness strategy but a reflection of 'rank-ordering' to explicitly or implicitly acknowledge the relationship between the speaker and hearer, as a 'relation-acknowledging device' (1988: 414). In other words, understanding where the speaker positions themselves in relation to other members matters. She underlined how different the Japanese notion of face is as follows:

> Since a person's self-image is not as an independent individual but as a group member having certain relations to others, [Japanese] concept of 'face' is [fundamentally different from that of Europeans], who define themselves as individuals, with certain rights and a certain domain of independence. (Matsumoto, 1988: 423)

Matsumoto's claim reflects the social norms and behaviours in which people are expected to act according to their relative rank in a group or society, rather than projecting a self-image of an independent individual.

Similarly, Gu (1990) alleged that the Chinese notion of negative face, in situations of offering, inviting and promising, is different from that assumed in the framework proposed by Brown and Levinson and that exercising politeness strategies is not just an interactional instrument but also a normative phenomenon (1990: 242). Mao (1994) explained that the Chinese concept of face does not privilege the 'self' as much as Brown and Levinson's definition of face does. Rather, it represents a self-image that is linked to the views of the community, not individuals' wants towards themselves. Chinese face thus emphasises the harmony of individual behaviours with the judgement of the community rather than individuals' desires (1994: 460).

Ide *et al.* (1992) investigated how the term 'polite' and 'friendly' is conceptualised as against their American counterparts. For American students, the term 'polite' was correlated closely with 'friendly'. By contrast, these two adjectives fell into far different dimensions among Japanese students when applied to cross-culturally equivalent situations. The Japanese adjective '*teineina* (polite)' involved the speaker's sense of distance towards the hearer, the expression of which is conveyed by honorifics. On the other hand, '*shitashigena* (friendly)' indicates the speaker's sense of intimate attitude, which is often associated with the use of informal style or additional final particles along with honorifics (the use of an additional final particle functions as shortening the psychological distance between the speaker and hearer, in other words, it is 'a marker of familiarity'). It was argued that the use of honorifics is conventionally appreciated, even in a friendly relationship.

As shown above, honorifics and a marker of familiarity co-occur in the same sentence. Ide (1989) claimed that the sequence of linguistic choice projects the 'relative rank' of the participants and the speaker's adherence to the social norms and behaviours expected by others. This, however, is slightly contradictory, because holding both contrasting nuances in one utterance can indicate mitigating an FTA towards the speaker. The informal style – a marker of familiarity – functions as softening the rigidness of the formality. Matsumoto (1988) and Ide (1989) explained the characteristics of the Japanese language system, arguing that 'choice' is almost obligatory when it is based on the social norm. Ide (1989: 230) proposed a term, *wakimae*, which is an aspect that Brown and Levinson neglected. The practice of polite behaviour according to social conventions is known as *wakimae* in Japanese. To behave according to *wakimae* is to show verbally and non-verbally one's sense of place or role in a given situation according to social conventions.

The term *wakimae* is translated as 'discernment' (Ide, 1989: 230). In contrast to the concept of 'face-wants' as desire, the discernment aspect is focused on acknowledging the roles and settings of the participants. Thus, honorifics are not used to raise the hearer or lower the speaker, as Brown and Levinson (1987: 178) proposed in their theory, but to acknowledge their respective roles. Ide *et al.* (1992) concluded that the term 'polite' was volition-based, involving an evaluation of linguistic behaviours, whereas the Japanese adjective '*teineina* (polite)' was discernment-based – *wakimae* – addressing differences of social rank, and that it seemed therefore to be difficult to assume equivalence of the key concepts for universal politeness.

2.2.1.1 Evaluations towards the criticisms

There have been numerous discussions over such issues of cultural variability (Fukushima, 2000; Holtgraves, 2005; Spencer-Oatey, 2007; Usami, 2002, 2008; Yin *et al.*, 2012). Usami (2002) raised questions against the early criticisms and pointed out that some East Asian scholars misleadingly criticised Brown and Levinson's (1987) politeness theory based on an analysis of the language rules, thereby confusing sociolinguistics with pragmatics (2002: 19). Usami (2002) focused on two aspects of the early criticisms of Brown and Levinson's politeness theory:

(1) The concept of face is primarily based on Western perspectives and values, and the concept in Brown and Levinson's theory is fundamentally different from that in Chinese or Japanese culture (Gu, 1990; Mao, 1994; Matsumoto, 1988); and
(2) Brown and Levinson's politeness theory does not account for principles of linguistic politeness rules in Japanese and Chinese, including the use of honorifics (Gu, 1990; Ide, 1989; Mao, 1994; Matsumoto, 1988).

Addressing the first criticism, Usami (2002) argued that it resulted from a misinterpretation of the concept of linguistic politeness, which Brown and Levinson defined 'operationally' (2002: 20). She claimed that their politeness theory does not deny the fact that every culture has different nuances and connotations for the respective terms of face and politeness (Brown & Levinson, 1987: 58). However, culture-specific connotations for Brown and Levinson's terms are not provided, which means it is likely to cause some confusion for the interpretations. The second criticism claimed that there is little room for any rational or voluntary strategy in languages such as Japanese which have pragmatically obligatory use of honorifics. However, researchers have reported that there is certainly strategic language use. Usami (2002) noted that, in languages that have honorific systems such as Japanese, maintaining the normative use of honorifics can be performed to save the hearer's negative face; thus, it can function as a form of negative politeness and can also be FTA by deviating from the normative use of honorifics. This analysis presupposes that, as long as people use honorifics, people at least do not threaten the hearer's negative face. Japanese speakers frequently observe 'Speech-Level Shifts' (this will be briefly explained in Section 2.3.3) that involve strategic alternation between use and non-use of honorifics within an interaction (Ikuta, 1983; Pizziconi, 2003; Usami, 1993).

Holtgraves (2005) noted that cultural differences may result in wider variability in politeness theory, which can be explained as 'high level of abstraction, in terms of variability in power and distance' (2005: 84). In order to examine the conceptualisation of face, Spencer-Oatey (2007) applied social psychologist Schwartz's (1992) universal framework of 'value constructs' which has been empirically validated and covers more than 60 countries (Schwartz, 1992; Schwartz & Bardi, 2001). People surveyed for the research rated the importance of a wide range of different values such as obedience, loyalty, honesty, success and freedom that shape principles in their lives. According to Spencer-Oatey, the framework is useful, partly because people's value judgements could be influenced by the relative importance of their value constructs (2007: 649), and partly because the framework allows researchers to re-consider Brown and Levinson's distinctions between negative and positive face. She suggested that Brown and Levinson's negative face could be included under 'self-direction', which is linked to independent thoughts and action-choosing, and also the value constructs of independence, freedom, curiosity and creativity. On the other hand, positive face could potentially be a reflection of all the other value compositions (Spencer-Oatey, 2007: 650). These perspectives offer a more comprehensive understanding of the notion of face in different cultures and a framework for analysis in a multidisciplinary approach.

The criticisms from East Asian perspectives have focused on describing cultural varieties of linguistic politeness and has emphasised cross-cultural comparisons of the social norms and their conceptualisations. Usami (2008) commented that this variation is undoubtedly an important issue and that a certain type of behaviour could satisfy and/or infringe the hearer's face in a certain culture. This is why politeness theory has been extensively utilised in the analysis of professional communication in many different cultures, including social and healthcare contexts. In recent years, there has been some agreement that Brown and Levinson's theory can, in fact, be applied to the study of politeness in modern standard Japanese (Fukada & Asato, 2004; Pizziconi, 2003; Spencer-Oatey, 2007). Usami (2002, 2008) has suggested that, when a study applies the theoretical framework of Brown and Levinson to an analysis of politeness at the discourse level rather than utterances, the comparison of politeness systems across cultures can be explained. Thus, it seems inappropriate to question Brown and Levinson's entire theoretical construct.

2.2.2 Discursive approaches to politeness

There has been important work that has advanced the understanding of politeness theory. Criticisms of Brown and Levinson's (1987) theory have dealt with the complexity of the theoretical construction, and the importance of clearer distinctions between common-sense (lay) and theoretical (technical) terms in politeness research (Eelen, 2001; Kadar & Haugh, 2013; Kasper, 1990; Locher & Watts, 2005; Vilkki, 2006; Watts, 2003). Central to these critiques is the argument that, although Brown and Levinson's work does not completely ignore context, the framework encourages the analyst to examine politeness only at the utterance level, relying on the immediate contextual history behind a certain conversation. Moreover, it does not account for situations in which face-threat mitigation is not a priority, such as aggressiveness or rudeness, which would hardly be judged as polite. The theory of politeness is further developed by the work of Locher and Watts (Locher, 2006; Locher & Watts, 2005; Watts, 2003). They claim that politeness is only part of 'relational work' that is inherent in all social interactions and that politeness itself is a discursive concept arising out of interactants' perceptions and judgements towards verbal behaviours. The theorists have drawn linguists' attention to the fact that the interpretation of utterances is not as clear as Brown and Levinson's theory allows for, particularly when considering polite behaviours, interpersonal relationships, status and sensitivity, which must be treated as interconnected dimensions (Mills, 2011). Regarding the notion of face, Watts (2003: 130) suggests that face-work is not necessarily associated with the attribution of politeness and that all human interaction consists of face-work of one kind or another, which may include linguistic politeness as only one of its aspects. The 'discursive approach to politeness' looks at a number of turns or over longer stretches of the interaction, considering the issue of context. Thus, it no longer focuses on the phrase or sentence level and does not define politeness as being inherent in the words used by the speaker. Locher and Watts (2005) state that what is polite or what is impolite should not be predicted by researchers, and instead, researchers should focus on 'the discursive struggle' in which interactants engage (2005: 9). Considering these aspects, theorists refer to Brown and Levinson's theory as an early model of politeness with the focus of the speaker's mitigation of FTAs. The second order of politeness, on the other hand, is located within theorists' revised understanding and theoretical conceptualisation of politeness and impoliteness, which benefits discursive approaches to politeness (Van der Bom & Grainger, 2015).

However, there have been debates on its feasibility in research application. It has been argued that, as a consequence of the move towards second order of politeness, the discursive approach has led to a question of the analyst-participant distinction in politeness research and how researchers can identify politeness or impoliteness without imposing analysts' understandings (Haugh, 2007); the conceptualisation of relational work casts uncertainty over its analytical utility in politeness research (2007: 300). In addition, Mills (2011) states that theorists' conceptualisation of politeness may not coincide with that expressed by native speakers in general. Although many theorists have agreed with these critiques of Brown and Levinson's framework, many politeness researchers have recently gone back to the classical work of Brown and Levinson's model in latest articles (Van der Bom & Mills, 2015; Ramani *et al.*, 2018). For the purpose of this study that takes into account the link between face aspects and patient/person-centred account, the discursive aspect of politeness is not central to the analysis. However, the communicative strategies observed in medical consultations can be qualified in terms of their interactional and cultural context (which is further discussed in Section 2.3). Brown and Levinson's work seems the most influential framework of face and politeness so far, and it certainly provides an important basis for the discussion of face-work in the older patient–physician interactions.

Although 'culture' is a wide-ranging concept, it will be especially relevant to this study to look at views of culture from social (cultural) anthropology. In the following sections, I will explore some features of culture variations with specific reference to the concept of face, namely, individualistic and collectivistic values, high-context and low-context cultures, referring to Hofstede *et al.*'s ([1991] 2010) scheme of culture and Scollon *et al.*'s ([1995] 2011) contextual considerations of culture and face. I will then briefly provide an overview of the notion of 'Speech Level Shift' with regard to the use of Japanese honorifics.

2.3 Contextual Consideration

2.3.1 Individualism and collectivism

Social psychologist Geert Hofstede (1991) first introduced a model of national culture dimensions in the first publication of *Cultures and Organizations: Software of the Mind* (Hofstede, 1991), which was based on his comprehensive studies of how people's values in the workplace are influenced by culture. Hofstede (1991: 5) described culture as 'mental programming', using the metaphor of computer programming.

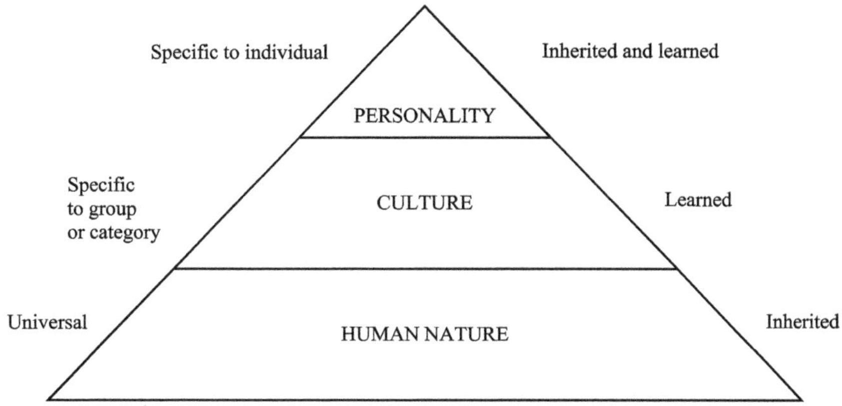

Figure 2.2 Three levels of uniqueness in mental programming (Hofstede *et al.*, [1991] 2010: 6)
Reproduced with the permission of the licensor.

He defined 'culture' as positioned within three levels of uniqueness in the relationship between (1) personality, (2) culture and (3) human nature; this is summarised below and in Figure 2.2. Culture is always a collective phenomenon, because it is at least partly shared with people who live or lived within the same social environment, which is where it was learned. Culture consists of the unwritten rules of the social game. It is the collective programming of the mind that distinguishes the members of one group or category of people from others (Hofstede, 1991: 5).

In this figure, culture is presented as learned, not innate, and also, culture is distinguished from human nature and personality. Under human nature, Hofstede (1991) included the abilities to feel fear, anger, joy and sadness as universal and inherited traits. Personality is also presented as learned and a unique personal set of mental programmes that are not necessarily shared with others.

Hofstede studied a large body of survey data about the values of people in more than 50 countries and developed the model of national culture dimensions. The model consists of six dimensions: 'power distance index', 'individualism versus collectivism', 'masculinity versus femininity', 'uncertainty avoidance index', 'long-term orientation versus short-term normative orientation' and 'indulgence versus restraint' (Hofstede *et al.*, [1991] 2010). The dimension of 'individualism versus collectivism' seems to be particularly important to this chapter, because it is strongly associated with the relationship between the notions of self and group and how this affects participants' communicative strategies. Oyserman *et al.* (2002) state that Hofstede's model is important because it organises cultural differences into overarching patterns that have expanded the body of cultural research.

Regarding the distinction between individualism and collectivism, Hofstede called 'individualist' those societies in which individuals are expected to take care of themselves and their immediate families. In contrast, he called 'collectivist' those societies in which individuals expect the members of a particular group to look after them out of loyalty. From this perspective, people in an individualistic culture often recognise the importance of self and independent responsibility, where social behaviour tends to be led by personal goals. Collectivistic cultures, on the other hand, stress values for group orientation, collaboration and conformity, where people are expected to be willing to maintain a relationship of membership. These individualistic-collectivistic dimensions reflect the position of a society in terms of whether 'self' of a member of a society is 'I' (with independent responsibility) or 'we' (with group harmony). Drawing on Hofstede, Triandis (1989) exemplified people in North and Western Europe and North America as displaying individualist traits; on the other hand, people in Asia, Africa and South America display elements of the collective self.

One must be careful, however, and avoid linking different discourses (shaped by social actions, participants and places) with broad categories of national or regional cultures. For example, in North America, which is characterised (classified) as an individualist culture in the claims above, people tend to show stronger interest in their community activities, compared to Japanese culture, which is considered collectivist (Inoue, 1997). Gudykunst *et al.* (1996: 530) mentioned that 'previous research demonstrates that when college students are sampled in Japan and the United States, Japanese college students often are more individualistic than college students in the United States'. Likewise, other different types of collectivism can also be interpreted as individualistic. Scollon *et al.* ([1995] 2011: 59) have claimed that 'whether one's orientation towards face is individualistic or collectivistic may have to do with one's age, gender, profession, or the contingencies of a particular situation as much as with one's regional or national culture, and people who share regional and national cultures may exhibit considerable variation in their politeness behaviour'.

Generational variation is also seen in individualist-collectivist terms. There are at least two theories that explain generational discourse variations. The first theory is the 'general subcultural theory', which focuses on the beliefs and social events of a given generation. The second theory is known as the 'life-cycle theory', which explains that people's behaviour will evolve and universally become more conservative and more collectivistic as they grow older, throughout the sequence of life events (Scollon *et al.*, [1995] 2011: 208). Although individualism is commonly assumed as the opposite of collectivism, there is evidence of categorisation of individualism and collectivism co-existing in every group (not necessarily within a culture but a group having something in common). Triandis (2001) commented that it should not be assumed that everybody in individualist cultures has all the characteristics of that culture, and vice versa; rather, it depends on the 'situation' because the 'situation' is a powerful predictor of the level of cooperation (Triandis, 2001: 912).

Another aspect highlighted by Triandis *et al.*'s early study (1986) is that family integrity and interdependence factors are important aspects of collectivism, and people in a collectivist culture tend to deal with strangers differently, compared to individualist cultures. This means that the identity of a group tends to be perceived differently between individualists and collectivists. Anthropologist Edward T. Hall (1976) defined group identity through developing a theory of 'high-/low-context' cultures and relevant communication patterns. I will look at this theory and the aspect of group harmony in the following section.

2.3.2 High context and low context

The theory of 'high context' and 'low context', as defined by Hall (1976), is widely recognised as a framework to capture cultural differences between societies. Hall illustrated this concept using a number of nationalities and considered Asian, Latin American and southern European societies to be 'high-context' cultures, whereas North American and northern European were considered low-context cultures. 'High-context' culture refers to societies where cultural customs and contextual aspects, such as background knowledge and settings of the communication, are not made explicit because most members of the group know implicitly what to think and what to convey to each other. Hall (1976: 79) pointed out that in high-context cultures, more information is conveyed in the non-verbal aspects of communication than in the verbal aspects. 'Low-context' culture, in contrast, indicates societies where cultural beliefs and background of the communication may need to be stated explicitly so that people coming into the cultural environment know how to behave. In other words, face-to-face interactions in high-context cultures are characterised by an extensive use of nonverbal elements, including gestures, silence and closeness. In contrast, low-context culture tends to be less physically animated, depending on the spoken words. In each culture, of course, there are specific individual differences in the need for 'contexting' – the process of filling in background data (Hall & Hall, 1990: 7).

One salient aspect is that Hall's concept provides a clear definition of these two key terms, which has been acknowledged and applied in cross-cultural research. At the same time, this definition has been criticised for leading to bipolarisation and overgeneralisation, or for representing 'older' classifications of national cultures that no longer apply (Kittler *et al.*, 2011). Scollon *et al.* ([1995] 2011: 40) oppose labelling whole 'cultures' in terms of high context and low context. For example, people tend to be low context in a court of law, where hearing and talking are made verbally explicit. This is because these are specific 'speech events' or 'situations' that require explicitness. Furthermore, in social situations such as dinner settings with family members and close friends, utterances include a high amount of meaning that is communicated non-verbally by reference to the context (2011: 41). Thus, these categories are not completely separable. The 'high-/low-context' distinction was initially applied to nationalities or language groups, but the concept has now also been applied to social communities, corporations, professions and situations.

Scollon *et al.* ([1995] 2011: 64) note that, in an individualistic context, the way of speaking to others is similar from situation to situation, since in each case, the identity of membership is being negotiated and developed within the situation of the discourse. On the other hand, in a collectivist context, many relationships are established from one's birth into a particular family in a particular place. These 'memberships' tend to take on a character along with special forms of discourse, which preserve the boundaries between insiders and outsiders.

As outlined in the previous chapter, the communication styles in Japan deeply rely on non-verbal aspects such as nods, fillers, postures and silence (Kita & Ide, 2009; Maynard, 1993), as well as on the system of honorifics. These aspects seem to be an inseparable set of communicative patterns that support relationship; thus, their use and the modes of address for ingroups and outgroups could be considered characteristic of a collectivistic context.

2.3.3 Japanese honorifics

The use of honorific expressions (polite forms) has been a well-researched area in language and communication studies in general. Many aspects of honorifics are encoded in the grammatical system and are rather difficult to avoid (Ide, 1989; Shibamoto-Smith, 2011). In verbal interactions, honorifics indicate the social relationship between speakers and hearers, or between participants and third parties involved in the context, as a way to show mutual respect. Two basic forms are the intent of respect and of humbleness, based on disparities in the ages, experiences and social roles of the speakers. For example, different forms of address are used to differentiate between formal and private occasions. This indicates that when the speaker uses respect forms, the hearer can recognise what sort of interpersonal relationship is intended by the speaker, such as their social rank in a professional situation and seniority in a group. Similarly, when honorifics are absent in social situations, the hearer recognises the friendly relationship specified by the speaker. 'Speech-Level Shifts' occur when the speaker is an active agent 'who strategically choose to use honorific or non-honorific forms to achieve their interactional goals' (Cook, 2011: 3658). The speaker makes a choice relying on his or her assumption as to whether the participants' age groups, responsibilities and occupational titles would be nearly equal to their own or not, or whether the speaker would like to communicate in total informal style (Cook, 2011).

Modern society is based on social groups where members accept each other as 'equal', compared to the traditional norms when honorifics were rigidly used in a fixed social hierarchy (Okushi, 1988). Usami (2002) analysed Japanese natural conversations between unacquainted people from the perspective of discourse-level politeness. She found that honorifics function more frequently as a stylistic choice than as a reflection of the actual relationship as was traditionally the case and that female subjects used more honorifics than males. This means that the historical tradition has now transformed into modern practice that appreciates mutual respect.

In 2007, the Agency for Cultural Affairs of the Government of Japan officially published guidelines on honorific expressions (Agency of Cultural Affairs, Governments of Japan, 2007). The guidelines mention that the use of honorifics should essentially be expressions chosen by the speaker, meaning that the speaker exercises independent judgement on each occasion. It proposed to classify Japanese honorifics into five functions:

(1) forms of respect (*sonkei-go*)
(2) forms of humbleness 1 (*kenjo-go 1*)
(3) forms of humbleness 2 with graciousness (*kenjo-go 2*)
(4) forms of politeness (*teinei-go*)
(5) forms of beautifying (*bika-go*)

These five functions can be summed up into three types: forms of respect, humbleness and politeness. The difference between the respect and politeness forms is linked to whether the participants' positions are differentiated or not. When using the form of respect (*sonkei-go*), the speaker does not position their own side as higher than the hearer. 'The speaker's side' does not only mean the speaker but also refers to anyone who belongs to the same group as the speaker, such as family members and colleagues. For example, the speaker addresses '*sensei* (doctor)' and uses the respect form '*irassharu* (to be)' instead of the informal style '*iru* (to be)', stating '*seisei ga irassharu* (the doctor is here). In this situation, the speaker uses a form of respect while maintaining a certain distance and placing the doctor in a higher position. If the participants' social positions are equal or nearly equal, the respect form can be used by both speakers. Forms of politeness (*teinei-go*), on the other hand, are generally used by all speakers in the interaction, regardless of the positioning. Using them is obligatory unless the speaker intends to choose an informal style. This is an important aspect, because it is reported that Japanese doctors tend to balance informal style and honorifics, rather than using honorifics throughout. This observation indicates that, at least to some degree, doctors attempt to create nearly equal relationships (Yoshioka *et al.*, 2008; Yoshioka & Shin, 2010).

The following section discusses empirical investigations of politeness research in medical encounters. I will then conclude this chapter by discussing the link between patient-centred communication (PCC) and face and politeness notion.

2.4 Empirical Work in Medical Encounters

Extensive empirical research has examined how verbal interaction shapes politeness in different healthcare settings and how conceptualisations of politeness are linked to professional practice. Previous studies cover a variety of healthcare-related workplaces, including hospital wards and elderly care homes. In terms of politeness strategies focusing on elderly care settings, several studies have been carried out in the US, Australia, England, Germany, South Africa, Sweden and Japan.

Makoni and Grainger (2002) explored the interactional strategies between caregivers and elderly residents in nursing homes in the UK and South Africa and compared the discourse of caring (e.g. bathing, getting up routines and lunchtime events). They found that there were a large number of similarities in these two settings, regarding the role of the institutional environment (the role of caregivers as service providers, and simultaneously as controllers). For example, positive politeness strategies such as expressing intimacy and sympathy were noticeably seen in the caring settings. An inherent tension potentially lies in these settings, in which 'the [act] of "caring" necessitates physically intrusive, embarrassing, or [painful medical procedures] which at the same time are intended to benefit the recipient of the care' (2002: 807). The authors pointed out that the physical act of caring involves threats to both negative and positive face that have to be redressed with positive politeness strategies (2002: 816). The strategies make sense because the care providers need to deal with such high levels of sensitivity in terms of embarrassing examinations and physical pain, in which they support the resident's positive face want by expressing intimacy and sympathy, as well as protecting negative face want.

Backhaus (2009) analysed interactions in an elderly care home in Japan, which took place in settings similar to that of the study above – bathing, getting up routines and lunchtime settings. Backhaus included a cross-cultural comparison with data from previous research in a German nursing home, a UK geriatric hospital ward and the caring institution in South Africa examined by Makoni and Grainger (2002). Backhaus found significant similarities in the use of positive politeness strategies in this cross-cultural comparison, such as giving praise, inclusive joking and exclusive joking. He noticed that these findings were in accordance with three characteristics of linguistic interaction in institutional elderly care proposed by Grainger (2004): (1) a conspicuous absence of talk, (2) the pervasiveness of task-oriented talk and (3) staff members' intentional or non-intentional emphasis on the frailty and helplessness of the residents (Grainger, 2004). Specifically, staff member's 'superlative talk' which involves the use of exaggerated praise (Lanceley, 1985: 130) was similarly observed in a nursing home in Germany, South Africa and the UK. Backhaus reported that the strategy of giving praise was not positively received when it was perceived as an expression of resident staff in an unequal power relation. This means that giving praise could be potentially perceived as excessive praise to the residents and could be taken overly personally. Backhaus (2009) observed that the power difference between caregivers and residents in Japan was shown by the staff's speech styles: staff addressed residents by their first name and mostly used informal style rather than honorifics. In addition, inclusive and exclusive joking without cooperation with residents was seen as a failure to create familiarity in the settings in Japan, South Africa and the UK, while joking could be effective in confirming an already established relationship between the staff and the resident (Backhaus, 2009). Joking is a basic technique of positive politeness for putting the hearer at ease or minimising FTAs (Brown & Levinson, 1987: 124). However, it can also be a way of asserting intimacy here. Using jokes, thus, seems to be a potentially risky conversation style when used by staff towards residents. Furthermore, similar issues have been raised regarding on-record strategies of positive politeness. In hospital settings, it was pointed out that positive politeness strategies – particularly, admiring, talking optimistically, sympathy and praise – may have different effects depending on the patients' face and that doctors often apply minimal use of honorifics and more use of informal style and local dialects to establish initial rapport with their patients (Tokuda *et al.*, 2008; Yoshioka *et al.*, 2008; Yoshioka & Shin, 2010).

Yoshioka *et al.* (2008) called the use of politeness strategies in clinical consultations *clinical politeness*, defining patients' positive face as 'the want to be understood, sympathised with and acclaimed by medical professionals, and the want to shorten the psychological distance with the professionals'. The patient's negative face is described as 'the want not to be disturbed, keep a psychological distance with the professionals, and the want to be treated politely by them' (Yoshioka *et al.*, 2008; Yoshioka & Shin, 2010). The methods used in their studies included discourse analysis of medical interviews between patients and physicians in a public hospital in Japan, follow-up interviews with the patients and physicians, and an online survey of physicians' views. They highlight the following results (Yoshioka *et al.*, 2008):

(1) Physicians tended to use positive politeness strategies, which often included 'using in-group identity markers' and 'being optimistic'.
(2) Both doctors and patients confirmed that non-hierarchical relationships and minimal levels of honorific use would be suitable to clinical consultations.

(3) Physicians using the same dialect as that of the patients were able to enhance the relationship with the patient. This also facilitated the patients' narrative and enabled doctors to collect much information from the patient.
(4) Such positive politeness strategies as 'exaggeration (e.g. interest, approval, sympathy)' and 'being optimistic' might affect the relationship negatively if the physician has missed the situation in which the patient find themselves and their face need.

These findings show two aspects: the physicians are aware that the patients prefer equal or nearly equal relationships and prefer to talk to their doctors using a minimum level of polite forms (honorifics). At the same time, physicians are also aware of the potential risk of missing the patient's face wants.

Yoshioka and Shin (2010) further examined clinical politeness strategies and identified 16 positive politeness strategies in the consultations, 15 of which were adopted from Brown and Levinson's politeness theory, and one additional strategy; this 16th positive politeness strategy was articulated as 'talk to patients avoiding an excessive level of polite forms to remove a sense of distance between doctors and patients' (2010: 40). Seven negative politeness strategies were also identified. The findings supported the discussions in the previous findings that (1) overuse of polite forms can have a detrimental effect on the doctor–patient relationship and (2) patients expected doctors to use more informal expressions than doctors had expected. Yoshioka and Shin (2010) concluded that the overuse of polite expressions can cause non-effective doctor–patient relationships, and the use of language directly reflects the psychological distance between them and affects their communication.

2.5 Conclusions

These strategic choices have been strongly related to acts of building rapport and relationships, the creation of trust and providing information, which are part of the key goals of PCC, and more broadly, related to patients' satisfaction. Since it has been suggested that PCC depends on identifying each patient's individual needs and expectations, it is profoundly to do with the notion of face. Considering face-work and rapport management in medical encounters is an important part of documenting the characteristics of the research context (Locher & Schnurr, 2017). The reason why the empirical studies above have chosen to apply Brown and Levinson's politeness theory to their analyses is because the theory is predominantly concerned with face-work and is efficient as an analytical framework for evaluating real-life clinical interactions between patients and professionals. While agreeing with criticisms made on the theoretical and scientific conceptualisation, Backhaus (2009) states that his analysis relied on Brown and Levinson's framework to a large extent because the model provides a helpful and well-established terminology for analysing linguistic interactions (2009: 57). Yoshioka *et al.* (2008) have not specified their reason for adopting Brown and Levinson's politeness theory in their papers; however, they note that the framework contains precise terminologies that allowed the Japanese researchers to define clear Japanese translations for equivalent terms. Taking into account these points of view, as well as the fact that this study also uses data from clinical settings in Japan and given the close compatibility between face and PCC dimensions, it has been deemed appropriate to use Brown and Levinson's concepts of face and politeness in this study too. In the construction of the analytical framework used in this book, PCC domains will be integrated with face aspects to analyse medical consultations.

3 Fieldwork and Data

Chapter 3 presents the details of the ethnographic fieldwork, the outline of participants and data, inclusion criteria, procedures of transcription and translation, and ethical considerations. This is followed by the general structure of the medical consultations I observed, and the development of the analytical categories to examine physician patient-centred communication (PCC) communicative acts in the authentic interactions. This chapter concludes with presenting a full illustration of the Face-PCC analytical framework.

3.1 Ethnography and Observational Fieldwork

Today, the term 'ethnography' encompasses a broader range of work; ethnographers do not necessarily observe events directly but may work with written documents or study audio or video recordings of social interactions (Silverman, 2014). Contemporary researchers share the idea that the term 'ethnography' is used broadly as the equivalent to the general application of qualitative methods (Hammersley, 1992; Silverman, 2014). This involves the explicit distinction made between 'observer' and 'participant' roles during the research activities. Gold (1958) conceptualised the research roles that be adopted in this approach as follows: (1) *Complete participant*, whose purpose in the field is not known to those whom the researcher observes, and whom the researcher interacts with as naturally as possible; (2) *Participant as observer*, whose role differs in the sense that the researcher and informants are aware that they have a 'field relationship'. The researcher will often spend many months or years working with the community, developing relationships and participating as well as observing; (3) *Observer as participant* is a researcher whose study may involve one-visit interviews and the emphasis is more on formal observation than participation. Gold (1958) pointed out that contact time is much briefer in this role than in the other two roles and can be quite superficial. Therefore, it is more likely for the researcher to misunderstand the informants or to be misunderstood by them; lastly, (4) *Complete observer* is a researcher whose physical presence is not involved, and who observes people in a way that makes it unnecessary for them to take the researcher into account. Studying written documents, audio or video recordings of social events or interactions would fit this research role. These four characteristics of participation mean that the researcher may be involved to various different degrees of field relationships, entailing different methodological concerns. As Gold pointed out, an observer-as-participant might be in a weaker position, because he or she takes only a quick dip into the field, which is likely to result in inadequate understanding and even miscommunication between the researcher and informants, due to shorter periods of contact time. A common criticism of ethnography is articulated by Hammersley (1992) when he argues that there are issues around the representation of social reality and an ambiguity between the researcher and social practice, which can lead to a lack of understanding of the local culture and practice.

Medical anthropologists have traditionally taken more of a participant-as-observer role observing the health beliefs and practices of a community or culture while being embedded in that community or culture to see 'what is going on' through their eyes. This has contributed to the development of the basics of contemporary 'observational studies' or 'fieldwork' in health research. Green and Thorogood (2018: 59) explain that in health settings, the term 'observational study' involves research designs in which there is some 'direct' observation of a site, talk or practice, without an intervention by the researcher. Observational designs have been frequently used to evaluate the real-life applicability of research evidence in health research, allowing the researcher to document a participant's social behaviour and to explore a specific situation (case) in its natural context. This implies that the researcher does not 'deliberately' intervene in the interaction of those being studied and that the data collected are naturally occurring in the setting being observed.

Fieldwork is also undertaken to gain a broader perspective on the health context, by considering the professionals' different experiences and the impact of these on their practice. Many health research projects involve both observation and participation in fieldwork. For example, Mondaca *et al.* (2018) conducted a six-month field study focusing on older adults' daily activities living in nursing homes, which included participation in activities. One of the authors positioned herself as a frequent guest in the nursing home and used narrative ethnography as a method to document the participants' informal and formal conversations, activities and archival materials; a corpus of fieldnotes was applied for the analysis. Their findings highlight the meaning of everyday activities in the institutional setting.

In another approach, Ottrey *et al.* (2020) conducted a four-month field study that involved observing hospital staff's mealtime practices, attitudes and beliefs in nutrition care across breakfast, lunch and dinner, combined with interviews and focus group discussions. These methods generated understanding of hospital staff's behaviours regarding how they cooperated with mealtime interventions (that seek to improve the food intake of patients) and the extent to which they recognised the values of supporting patient care. These different roles, i.e. as an 'observer' or a 'participant', can be equally valuable as core activities in the field.

I adopted a participant-as-observer role, spending six months with participants observing real-life clinical interactions. This enabled me to select a set of case studies in particular settings that would enable me to conduct an in-depth exploration. I attended the staff meetings in the respective clinics before the timetables of consultations were drawn up, and I travelled to patients' homes with health professionals in the same car, as well as observing and audio recording medical consultations. My fieldwork also included post-observation interviews with physician participants. This routine was repeated for four to five days a week during the period of fieldwork, fitting in with the timetables of the respective participating clinics. All these activities enhanced my understanding of the professionals' perspectives, and the institutional and local political situations.

3.2 Naturally Occurring Data

The primary focus of my observational fieldwork in Japan was the verbal elements of participants' communication. While fieldnote-taking was essential in recording contextual data, making audio recordings of the actual medical consultations was the most appropriate means to collect concrete empirical evidence. Thus, the audio-recorded data and accompanying observational notes (e.g. keywords, actions of who, where, when and my initial interpretations) were the raw data collected during my period of observation. Data that derive from situations that exist independently of the researchers' intervention is called *naturally occurring data* (Golato, 2003; Potter, 2002). Kasper (2000) reviews the advantages of utilising naturally occurring talk: researchers can observe native (and non-native) speakers in their social roles (e.g. in this study, the health professionals, patients and families). In the field of pragmatics, researchers can capture the variability that reflects the social speech events, and the strategic, actional and linguistic choices by which the speaker attempts to reach their communicative goals (Kasper & Dahl, 1991). Golato (2003) notes that making audio recordings enables the researcher to study how language is organised and realised in 'natural' settings. However, it has been pointed out in the existing literature that speech acts may not always occur 'naturally' (Kasper, 2000; Potter, 2002). In criticism of the analysis of naturally occurring data, it has been claimed that the presence of the researcher may alter the normal course of the interaction being studied. In addition, the presence of the recording equipment may become intrusive or an obstacle. Potter (2002) discusses the distinction between natural and contrived data:

> I do not see this as an injunction to find data that are 'unbiased' – that would be a very traditional notion of data and purity. Rather I see it as

> highlighting the researcher's central place in the production of conventional research data, and highlighting the virtue of material where the researcher's active role is minimized. (Potter, 2002: 539)

The notion of 'natural' here can be seen as rather limited – it is rather, *naturalistic* data (Potter, 2002), because research participants may consequently modify their actions in a variety of ways. Tannen ([1984] 2005) notes that, as long as participants are aware of the presence of the recorder, their talk is not natural; however, there is evidence that participants often forget about the recorder, which is what happens in her studies (Tannen, [1984] 2005: 44). In health research settings, Epstein *et al.* (2005) argue that the methodological problem arising from collecting data from spontaneous interactions is that both physicians and patients are likely to modify their behaviours when they know that they are being observed. By contrast, Sarangi (2010b) points out that professionals and patients are used to having third-party observers and therefore, he argues, the presence of the researcher is less of an issue. Although this methodological issue has been much debated, it does seem that participants are likely to perform naturally in a clinical setting overall. Furthermore, as long as the researcher recognises these limitations, it is possible to minimise the obstacles by considering where to position the recording equipment or make a recording without the observer being present in the same room. Therefore, it can be said that naturally occurring talk is authentic because it is spontaneous. Moreover, the nature of naturally occurring data should be distinguished from *researcher-provoked data* (Silverman, 2014) such as research interviews, focus groups, role plays or any experimental interactions which do not exist apart from the researcher's intervention. In light of these considerations, my priority was to reduce the potential impact of my presence to a minimum. More specifically, I had a short general conversation with each participant prior to explaining the project, and then immersing myself into the conversation between the participants rather than taking fieldnotes on my own.

3.3 Ethical Approval

This study was approved by the International Development Research Ethics Committee at University of East Anglia on 31 July 2017, and by the Ethics Committee of Tokyo-Hokuto Health Co-operative Association on 2 February 2018. Permission to conduct the observations was sought from the physician participants and the upper management of the clinics in Japan; thus, no formal or otherwise governmental approval that falls under the Ethical Guidelines for Medical and Health Research Involving Human Subjects in Japan was needed for this study. Data collection involved fieldnote-taking and audio recordings on the approval of all parties including the professionals, patients and their families where applicable.

3.4 Field Sites

The field research took place from December 2017 to May 2018. Data collection involved visiting eight clinics located in populated wards around the centre of Tokyo: Arakawa-ward, Adachi-ward, Bunkyo-ward, Toshima-ward, Nerima-ward, Nakano-ward, Setagaya-ward and lastly, Yokohama city, which is an hour and a half away from Tokyo.

There are 23 wards within the Tokyo area, and each ward is accessible in 15 to 20 minutes by train or metro, meaning that the wards are very closely situated to each other. There, the Tokyo Metropolitan Government handles administrative policies and services, but there are significant differences in social welfare and support for elderly care, occupations and household incomes of the residents, as well as the town landscapes and scenery in the wards. In the setting of physician in-home consultations, the doctor leads a medical team that generally includes a nurse and other staff who assist the doctor, nurse and patient. They visit the patient's home every two weeks or once a month, depending on the patient's medical needs, which costs a monthly management fee, and the patient incurs the cost of the service. To be entitled to the service, the patient must be unable to travel to a local outpatient clinic, although there are also several patients who refuse to go to a hospital or clinic. The typical daily timetable for physician consultations can be illustrated as follows: the morning timetable is scheduled between 9am and 12pm (four to five patients in the morning) and between 1pm and 5pm (six to seven patients in the afternoon). After the medical team has done the preparation, a contracted driver takes them to each patient's house by car. One consultation is expected to last approximately 20 minutes. Each clinic has 150 to 200 enrolled patients, and five to seven physicians are stationed to conduct home visits. At the same time, most of the physicians also practice in outpatient services in the clinic on different days.

3.5 Healthcare System in Japan

The Japanese healthcare system is regulated by the administration of the Ministry of Health, Labour and Welfare. Most healthcare providers are private institutions; 85% of the hospitals and 95% of the clinics are privately owned. It is compulsory for all citizens to be enrolled in a health insurance programme. An insurance card is issued to all citizens after enrolment, and the beneficiaries are guaranteed access to healthcare providers from general practitioners to specialists. Patients are responsible for being charged a part of the medical costs: 20% of the costs for people aged 70 and over, 30% for people aged under 70, and 0% in publicly funded health care. Both the public and private healthcare providers have been incentivised to prescribe drugs and tests because they receive medical fees based on fee-for-service for each prescription or test, rather than time spent with patients.

The need to enrich and disseminate medical and nursing care is made even more urgent due to a further social issue. It has been proposed that beds used by long-term hospitalised older patients in large hospitals should be converted into long-term care facilities. The purpose of this proposal is to reduce 'social hospitalisation' among older patients who do not require medical treatment, yet do not leave the hospital due to their incapability of living at home. This has also caused a problem for the younger generation who feel forced to take care of their parents at home and tend to leave their workplaces to look after parents, which affects the dynamism of the economic and social factors of care (Watanabe *et al.*, 2018). This situation further strengthens the needs to investigate the values that in-home medical consultations offer.

3.6 Gatekeepers

Before illustrating the research participants, I must mention about the gatekeepers who allowed me to gain access to the medical teams and their patients. Gatekeepers can support or limit access depending on their professional opinions or ideas regarding the feasibility and validity of the research. In this study, the primary gatekeeper was a family physician with 15 years' experience. I have known this doctor since 2016, when I was writing my MA dissertation on doctor's empathy expressed for patients in medical interviews at University of East Anglia. Before meeting the doctor, I was focusing on systematic literature review on clinical empathy in the medical education context, hoping that I could collect more information about textbooks used in medical school and guidelines on the aspects of showing empathy in primary care settings. My supervisor encouraged me to find and ask local experts about the subject matter and not to hesitate to ask them questions. I sent an email to medical school in Tokyo with introducing myself and the possibility of hearing some information about what students are taught regarding empathy in the educational context. One school replied to me, and they offered some documents such as syllabus and seminar materials, and they also invited me to come and observe a seminar, which was a training session for simulated patients who attended for the Objective Structured Clinical Examination (OSCE). In June, after the semester ended, I flew from the UK to Tokyo and visited the medical school to sit in the seminar. There, I was introduced to a doctor, who had researched clinical interactions with patients and empathy among medical students, and later became the gatekeeper in this study. The secondary gatekeeper was an experienced family physician, and I was introduced to the doctor for the first time during my preliminary fieldwork in August 2017. He had specialised in patient–doctor communication research while having over 20 years of practical experience in primary care as well. He generously offered to become the second gatekeeper of local contacts during my fieldwork. It turned out that the icebreaker with these gatekeepers were our curiosity and enthusiasm on the similar research topics around patient–doctor interactions. Some experts offer help, even when you do not have a personal or direct connection with the person or institution.

The first crucial step was these gatekeepers' decisions on who to select and recruit as physician participants for this study, following seeking permission from all physician participants and the upper management of clinics.

3.7 Physician Participants

Through these two gatekeepers, their colleagues, who had years of practice ranging from 10 to more than 20 years, were asked whether they were interested in participating in this study. The majority of doctors who engaged in in-home medical consultations were board-certified family physicians, who are at least 10 years post-qualification. This means that the context of physician in-home consultations for older adults primarily requires experienced doctors with more than 10 years of practice. Thus, I was not able to include junior doctors who normally establish their early careers in hospital settings. Two resident doctors participated in this study, as they were assisting some consultations as part of their training programme.

Prior to a face-to-face meeting with potential physician participants, I first explained, by email, that this was a study of authentic consultations between an older patient and a doctor, as well as the patient's family, where applicable, and that I would sit in the consultation with the medical team, observe and collect audio recordings with permission from all the participants. After securing their agreement, I visited each doctor to have a face-to-face meeting, discussed the selection criteria for patient participants and relevant information about the patients' characteristics.

Eight physicians (five males and three females) participated in this study. I obtained written consent forms from all these physicians. The outline are included in the list of physician participants in Table 3.1.

The consultations involved other health professionals. In D1 and D3's consultations, the medical team included a doctor and a nurse. In D2's consultations, two resident physicians (trainees) attended and conducted a physical examination. For D4, D5, D7 and D8, the medical team consisted of a doctor, a nurse and an assistant whose role was to assist the logistics and type up patients' records. For D6, the team consisted of one or two doctors and an assistant, and the consultation was conducted by the doctor herself alone or with her colleague doctor. In addition, a professional role, a *care manager* is responsible for managing an individual's care service plan based on the client's situation, and care managers often attended their patients' medical consultations.

Table 3.1 A list of physician participants

Code	Gender	Age group, period of practice	Expertise	Average duration of consultation
D1	Male	40–44, 17 years	Family physician	14.5 minutes
D2	Male	50–54, over 20 years	Family physician	17.2 minutes
D3	Male	35–39, 14 years	Family physician	13.3 minutes
D4	Female	35–39, 13 years	Family physician	22 minutes
D5	Female	55–59, over 20 years	Family physician	17.8 minutes
D6	Female	40–44, 9 years	Family physician	27.7 minutes
D7	Male	30–34, 10 years	Psychiatrist	17.5 minutes
D8	Male	35–39, 12 years	Diabetologist	12.8 minutes

3.8 Patient Participants

For the recruitment of patient participants, I asked the doctors to select actual patients aged 65 and over who required a light level of support or care for daily activities and used the home visit service. They were confirmed to have the mental capacity to make rational decisions. We ensured that each patient participant cognitively understood the research objectives and agreed to anonymously take part in research (or with the patient's family's agreement where applicable). This was equivalent to Support Levels 1 and 2 or less and Care Level 1 out of 5 in the nationally standardised needs-certification system (Ministry of Health, Labour and Welfare, 2016). These certifications are given by the committee of municipal governments on the basis of the family physician's opinions and medical investigation results. The framework is helpful to set the guideline between us. However, at the point of data collection, patients' understanding and ability to participate needed further checked by consulting physician participants or their families where applicable. These consultations were made separately with the relevant caring parties so as to avoid a situation in which patients might have felt obliged to participate and abide by their doctors or family members' assessments. The recruitment process was as follows:

(1) The doctor identified eligible patients for this study from his or her patient list.

(2) When visiting the patient's house, the doctor gave the patient documents about this study, explained its objectives and the fact that participants would be anonymised and then asked if the patient would like to take part.
(3) If the patient agreed to participate, the doctor informed me of the timetable that included the patient's consultation.

I was allowed to observe the consultation with the same patient multiple times during the fieldwork. In some cases, I also attended other patients' consultations who had not initially been selected as participants but who allowed me to observe without recording. This happened when the medical team allowed me to join them at the last minute, and the patient and family members also allowed me to be present during the consultations. This (changeable context of timetable and observers) was not considered as abnormal, because it was frequently the case that additional resident physicians or other staff joined a scheduled consultation at a short notice, so the patients were informed in advance about having extra observers in their consultations.

As a result, I conducted observations of 74 patients. A total of 40 older patients (26 females and 14 males) agreed for recording their consultations. In terms of their socioeconomic profile, most of the patients can be categorised as belonging to the middle or upper middle class; they can afford to use multiple private care services, such as doctor or dentist home visit, nurse home visit, bathing service, day-care centre, carers and short stays in care homes. Table 3.2 shows the age distribution of the 40 older patients. The majority were aged between 80 and 94 years, and gender distribution was roughly 65% female and 35% male.[1]

Twelve out of the 40 patient participants had mild cognitive impairments and/or dementia in their early stages. In each case, the doctor confirmed that the patient understood information of the study, understood what was happening in the consultation and understood their right to

Table 3.2 Patient participant ages

Age group	*Female*	*Male*	*Total number*
65–69	0	1	1
70–74	3	1	4
75–79	2	1	3
80–84	6	3	9
85–89	4	3	7
90–94	8	3	11
95–99	3	2	5
	26	14	**40**

withdraw from the study at any moment. In light of the doctors' opinions, I confirmed that data collection in consultations with these patients was appropriate, and I made sure to obtain both the patient's and family member's agreement to participate.

Directly after each recording, I compared the audio data with fieldnotes and illustrated an overview of the general structure of the consultation and its main features. After this process, further considerations were taken into account regarding these 12 patients. I noticed that family member-doctor interactions were predominant in these consultations, and the doctor's facilitative responses were less frequent. It is reported that the nature of dementia consultations differs from those with patients who have stable cognitive capacity (Katsuno, 2005; Zaleta & Carpenter, 2010). In addition, it could be difficult even for the experienced doctors to assess whether these patients with dementia truly understood their right to withdraw if they became confused or uncomfortable during the course of the consultation with multiple participants. Considering these reasons and the research protocol for examining physician communicative acts, the consultations involving these 12 patients should be considered separately from those of the 28 other older patients who were cognitively in a stable condition. Therefore, the linguistic analysis of PCC acts primarily focuses on the consultations with the 28 older patients, due to differences in the nature of the consultations. However, the interactions with 12 patients with dementia and their families are discussed regarding the home and family context for the next chapters.

3.9 The Sample

Of the 28 patients, exactly half of them, i.e. 14 patients, attended their consultations on their own without the physical presence of a family member, and the rest of the 14 patients included their family members in their consultations. According to this distinction, I divided them into two groups: *Consultations A* for patients attending on their own, and *Consultations B* for patients attending with their families and/or friend or neighbour. Having an extra person in the consultation could result in different interactional barriers, connections and power relationships in the decision-making process (Vedel *et al.*, 2016).

There is an overall predominance of female participants at 60%. Below, the list of the participants in Consultations A is shown in Table 3.3, and the list of the participants in Consultations B is shown in Table 3.4.

The average duration of Consultations A was 18.4 minutes, whereas Consultations B lasted on average for 18.5 minutes: 14.4 minutes for the five male doctors and 22.6 minutes for the three female doctors. The average duration involving the three experienced doctors (with over 20 years' experience) was 16.8 minutes, while it was 18.4 minutes for the five younger physicians (less than 14 years' experience). Female doctors had

Table 3.3 A list of consultations with older patients attending on their own

Case number	Code, gender, age group	Duration of consultation (minutes)
01	P1, F, 95-99	19
02	P3, M, 90-94	16.1
03	P6, F, 90-94	17.1
04	P11, F, 90-94	24
05	P13, F, 80-84	26.3
06	P14, M, 65-69	12
07	P15, M, 80-84	20.8
08	P16, F, 85-89	16
09	P18, F, 80-84	11.1
10	P23, F, 70-74	36.5
11	P27, M, 80-84	10.1
12	P30, F, 85-89	14.7
13	P33, F, 70-74	19
14	P38, M, 85-89	15.5

Table 3.4 A list of consultations with older patients attending with their families

Case number	Code, gender, age group	Family member presenting	Duration of consultation (minutes)
15	P5, F, 85-89	Daughter	22.5
16	P7, F, 85-89	Daughter, neighbour	42.8
17	P17, M, 90-94	Son	15.1
18	P19, F, 80-84	Daughter	13.8
19	P20, F, 80-84	Husband	14.1
20	P21, M, 80-84	Wife	13.7
21	P22, F, 90-94	Brother, wife	26.2
22	P24, F, 90-94	Daughter	11.1
23	P25, F, 90-94	Husband	28.8
24	P31, M, 95-99	Daughter	15.5
25	P32, M, 70-74	Wife	15
26	P34, M, 85-89	Wife	19
27	P36, M, 75-79	Wife, daughter	10
28	P37, F, 70-74	Husband, daughter	11.3

more sociable conversations (small talk including non-medical discussions and affective statements) with the patient and family than male doctors, and the gender difference in the duration of consultations was seven minutes on average.

3.10 Fieldnotes and Recording Procedures

Fieldnotes (written notes) were made to keep track of the timetable, the patient's information, the room layouts, participants' sitting positions, topics discussed and other details about my actions in the field. Notes were made right after the interactions in order not to disturb the naturally occurring conversations. Regarding participants' noticeable gestures, I kept notes at the same time as the observations and audio recordings.

All recordings in the medical consultations were conducted according to the procedures described below:

(1) The medical team arrived at the patient's house, and the doctor introduced me to the patient and the family member where applicable. At this point, the patient roughly knew who I was and why I was visiting.
(2) I briefly explained what I would do while following the information of the research objectives and consent form. I asked if I could take an audio recording, gaining oral consent by audio recording after confirming their agreement. The audio recorders were turned on after this point. I was present as an observer and did not intervene at any point during the consultation.
(3) The recording was turned off when the doctor closed the consultation, and the medical team headed towards the entrance of the house.

3.11 Interviews as Researcher-provoked Data

Post-observation interviews with six physicians were also conducted. The purpose of the one-to-one interviews with the physician participants was to explore the doctor's professional background and individual differences related to their communication styles so as to capture any relevant information about contextual and practices in the analysis. Their individual differences include their background, training sites, their expertise, career path and the patient groups they often see, and how long and where they had been trained. In order to establish the route they had taken from their medical education through to the current point where they worked as a primary care physician, I conducted semi-structured one-to-one interviews with six of the eight physician participants, after observing their consultations. I was not able to interview the other two physicians. Timetables were not entirely regular, and it was difficult for some of the participants to find additional time before or after their consultation schedules that often changed on the day. When they informed me of extra availability for one-to-one interview, I visited the doctor on a different day that suited them.

Each interview lasted between about 40 and 60 minutes. I selected the method of the semi-structured interview, which is the most common form of interviewing in health research, as analysts can work effectively from having a predetermined list while also probing for details (Kelly, 2010). I started with the introductory question: 'Since graduating from medical school, has your communication style towards patients changed? If so, how and why?' Based on their responses, the next topics expanded. The following questions are examples I prepared for the overall areas of the interview. Note that I was not necessarily able to ask all these questions in the interviews; rather, the respective topics were follow-up questions based on the doctors' narratives.

- Could you tell me which classes or workshops were useful for you to learn medical interview skills or communication skills with patients?
- Are explanations about the patient-centred approach in educational material appropriate enough, regarding actual practice?
- What sort of factors do you think would affect the individual differences of doctors in their communication styles with patients? For example: expertise, locations, etc.
- Do non-verbal behaviours of communication have any influence on verbal communication styles during the consultations?

The interview became more in-depth as I proceeded with these narrative-based questions, leading to relatively long narratives of the patients' stories I observed in most cases. This interviewing style may not be strictly semi-structured, but the aim of the one-to-one interviews with physician participants was to obtain an insight into the context of their transition from being a medical student to becoming a doctor in the current field, through additional training and/or experiences. This provided robust information regarding what brought the doctors to the individual interactional styles I observed in the consultations.

3.12 Transcription Procedures

I manually transcribed the audio files of the consultations and one-to-one interviews into a Word document. The transcribed data were then fully anonymised by removing any identifiable information such as names of persons, places or locations. The modern writing system of Japanese, *Kanji-Kana-majiri* was applied, which is a combination of Chinese characters and Japanese *kana* symbols. The advantage of this writing system is that it facilitates the quick review and comprehension of a large amount of transcripts by a native Japanese-speaking analyst.

The Jefferson system of transcription notation of conversation analysis (Jefferson, 2004) was then applied to the transcribed data. The list of symbols employed in this study is included in Appendix 9.1. Conversation analysis captures not only what is said but also details of how the multiple participants build speech actions and respond to the action of others (Hepburn & Bolden, 2013), which can be based on social and cultural aspects of the interaction. Annotating the transcripts in this way provided the foundation for the analysis of 'what' and 'when' the participants expressed.

3.13 Translation Procedures

The utterances were translated as a three-line interlinear gloss, which consists of the original source text in Japanese in the first line, a morpheme-by-morpheme (lexical gloss) of the original text in the second line and an idiomatic translation in the third line.

Example of the three-line interlinear gloss:

Case 1

13 D: <u>滑</u>ったの?
slip
Did you <u>slip</u>?

14 P: 氷のちょう[ど,
ice just
I was just on ice,

15 D: [あ : : 次の次の日が一番カチカチになったもんね.
寒かったもんね, マイナス４度になった日だよ, 多分.
aha next day most frozen
was cold minus four degree Celsius day probably
Ah, the street was frozen that day, two days after the snowing.
It was freezing. I guess we had –4°C that day.

Cross-cultural studies involving Japanese participants sometimes add Romanised Japanese (*Romaji*) into a gloss, which uses English alphabets to phonetically write Japanese, instead of the word-for-word translation. I applied the morpheme-by-morpheme (lexical gloss) for the second line, instead of Romanised Japanese, because it still keeps the original word order the same as the Romanised one, and the reader can see differences in syntax between Japanese and English and how original words and structures match those of the idiomatic translations. Alternatively, a four-line interlinear gloss including the source text, Romanised Japanese, word-for-word and idiomatic transitions could provide further transparency. However, a four-line gloss for each utterance would be an overload and distract the reader. It would also make it difficult to see the course of the conversations.

For its idiomatic translation in the third line, I tried to avoid translating literally but rather endeavoured to keep the original meaning and function of the speaker's message, as well as making the necessary grammatical and lexical adaptations. For example, the phrase in Japanese *'Please teach…'* has a broader meaning such as *'(Can I) have…'* or *'Tell (me)…'*, whereas, in English, the word 'teach' is used to convey the meaning of instructions or how to do something. Furthermore, the grammatical subject is very often omitted in Japanese. Thus, in the English translation, the missing subject is assumed from the functional meaning of the whole sentence. I also made sure that the lexical gloss of the original language accurately corresponded to the English vocabulary, based on the online Oxford Learner's Dictionaries.

In this book, however, the lexical gloss is omitted in order to improve the readability of the example text and make it easier to follow the conversations, as well as conceding to the space of this book. All the extracts presented in this book consists of the idiomatic translation for the first line and the original text for the second line of each example as follows:

Case 1

13 D: **Did you slip?**
滑ったの?

14 P: **I was just on ice,**
氷のちょう[ど,

15 D: **Ah, the street was frozen that day two days after the snowing. It was freezing. I guess we had −4°C that day.**
[あ：：次の次の日が一番カチカチになったもんね.
寒かったもんね, マイナス４度になった日だよ,多分.

All the translations were reviewed by a professional translator. I then revised the translations again, considering the comments made by the reviewer. The English translations were checked by an English native speaker. The transcription notation of conversation analysis (e.g. underlines, < >, [ ]) are also transferred from the source text onto the same parts of the idiomatic English translation. However, due to differences in the languages, the reproduction is only approximate.

3.14 Step 1: Consultation Phases

By transcribing each consultation closely, I first established a general structure of the in-home medical consultations in the data. In the consultations, the doctors signposted each stage with clear indication, which allowed me to see the phases and specific communicative skills used in each phase. This suggests an interesting correlation between the timing of the consultation and the frequency of PCC, when a specific PCC act can happen more often. For example, the first phrase included brief greetings and social talk to establish rapport, starting with *'Good morning/afternoon'* or *'It's nice weather today.'* The second phase began with a doctor's enquiry after checking the patient's record, *'How are you today?'* or *'How's your back pain?'* with follow-up questioning. The third phase, the physical examination, was conducted with statements asking permission to touch the patient's body, as in *'let me listen to your heart sound.'* The fourth phase, when prescriptions were discussed, typically started with *'Today, I will give you…'*, and the final phase included administrative tasks such as schedules for the next month, as in *'I will visit you in two*

Table 3.5 Consultation phases indicated by doctor's signposting

Phases	Sub-phases	Examples of doctor's signposting from the corpus
Phase 1	• Greetings	*'Good morning/afternoon.'* *'It's nice weather today.'* *'Thank you in advance.'*
Phase 2	• Topic initiation • Enquiry to gather information	*'How are you, father/mother?'* *'Isn't there any change?'* *'The other day, you had blood in your urine again, hadn't you?'*
Phase 3	• Physical examination	*'Shall I start the physical examination then?'* *'Well, let me listen to your heart sounds'*
Phase 4	• Prescription • Explanation • Planning and shared decision-making	*'Then, you still have some antibiotics left for four days, right?'* *'Then, today I won't give a prescription. Is it okay with you?'* *'Well, you have the numbness, but overall, I think you are in good condition. Here's your prescription.'*
Phase 5	• Closing • Administrative tasks: schedules and bills	*'Let's see how it goes. Your back pain might improve when it gets warmer. Let's make a judgement while looking at it.'* *'We are scheduled to come on 2nd April next time. I will see you then.'*

weeks.' The general structure of the consultations seems almost identical to the ideal structure, defined as the basic framework by the Calgary-Cambridge Guide. Table 3.5 shows the phases of the consultations and examples of doctor's signposting. Overlapping phases can also be identified by the contents of the topics, as summarised in Table 3.6.

3.15 Step 2: Face-PCC Analytical Framework

The consultation transcripts were manually coded to extract the PCC-relevant features and to identify correlations between the data and the PCC communicative domains defined by Epstein *et al.* (2005). This process allowed me to test what PCC-relevant communicative strategies are used (or not) and to see what indications of PCC, or potentially non-PCC, can be generated to further explore the speakers' linguistic forms in the analysis. Exploration of the patient's problems by the physician and the patient's expressions of concerns and feelings are particularly noticeable throughout the whole consultations. In order to keep the data manageable and maintain the focus on PCC communciative acts, I narrowed down the coding categories to cover the general phases of the consultations as seen in Section 3.14 *Step 1: Consultation phases*, including: (1) the beginning, (2) information gathering, (3) medication planning and (4) the closing of the consulation.

I adopted the terminologies of Communication Process Skills from the Calgary-Cambridge Guide that strictly follows the evidence from analysis of a wide range of healthcare situations and a set of doctor's desirable

Table 3.6 Consultation phases by contents derived from the preliminary analysis

Phases	Content
Greetings	The medical team arrived at the patient's house, and the doctor introduced me to the patient, and the family member where applicable. Since the patient and the doctor have known each other for months/ years, greetings or phrases occurring at this phase were brief.
Topic initiation	There were several patterns: (1) The medical team checked the patient's vital signs (body temperature, pulse rate, respiration rate, blood pressure) while asking general enquiries; (2) After spending a few minutes checking the patient's record, the doctor asked about appetite, meals (what and when), the condition of bowel movement, weight, fever (especially in January and February, flu was widespread; thus, the topic of fever was frequent).
Physical examination	If the medical team had a nurse or assistant, he or she checked vital signs, measured weight and the doctor listened to the heart. If necessary, the team delivered minor treatments, e.g. changed bandages, checked wounds, bruises, sprains, etc. The doctor's physical examination could be conducted either at the beginning or middle of the consultation.
Prescription	Commonly, prescriptions were discussed in-depth. Questions the doctor might ask included if the patient had problems taking medicine, whether it worked. Doctors might explain the medication's advantages and disadvantages and the possibility of changing amount/kinds of medicine. If a patient's family attended, this discussion was mainly between them and the doctor.
Planning/ Schedules	Occasionally, a blood test or hospital visit was planned. Schedules for the next month were discussed at the end of the consultation; this could often be a closing utterance.
Personal issues/ Closing	Patients and/or their family tended to relate a personal story or tale about living with the disease after the consultation was done. In some cases, hot drinks such as tea or coffee were offered. The medical team's schedule was usually busy and packed; hence, they often had to leave in a hurry.

communication skills, and the skills were tagged in the corpus. The relevant physician communicative skills in the data were then captured.

The skills were re-conceptualised in terms of the linguistic pragmatic notions of face and politeness – specifically, Brown and Levinson's (1987) classical politeness model. This allowed for the analysis of the occurrence of the doctor's communication skills with reference to their pragmatic functions and the specific context of culture that characterised the in-home medical consultations. I applied the definitions of positive and negative face as developed by Brown and Levinson (1987) to the physician communication skills. The PCC-relevant categories were then classified into the face aspects, based on the most relevant pragmatic form of the category, as Face-PCC analytical categories, as shown in Figure 3.1. In each category, short examples extracted from my data set are provided for illustration purposes.

I. ***Attends to Patient's Positive Face***

a. Identifies issues that the patient wishes to address

1. INITIAL GENERAL REMARKS [GR]
2. GRADUALLY MOVES FROM OPEN TO CLOSED QUESTIONS [OtoC]
3. [Potentially non-PCC] SEQUENCE OF CLOSED QUESTIONS AT THE BEGINNING [SeC]

b. Actively listens to the patient

1. REPETITION, PARAPHRASING AND INTERPRETATION [Lis]
2. [Potentially non-PCC] INTERRUPTION [Itr]

c. Displays empathy and acceptance

1. UNDERSTANDING AND APPRECIATION OF THE PATIENT'S FEELINGS [Und]
2. EXPRESSIONS OF POSITIVE REGARD [PR]
3. SILENCE AS EMPATHIC ANTICIPATION [Sil]
4. [Potentially non-PCC] BEING JUDGEMENTAL [Jud]

II. ***Attends to Patient's Negative Face***

a. Works towards shared decision-making

1. SHARING UNDERSTANDING [SU]
2. SHARING THINKING [ST]
3. OFFERING SUGGESTIONS [OS]
4. [Potentially non-PCC] NO SHARED DISCUSSION [NoSD]

b. Leaves space for the patient

1. OPEN QUESTIONS THAT OCCUR THROUGHOUT THE SESSION [OQ]
2. CHECKING FOR UNDERSTANDING [CU]
3. [Potentially non-PCC] DIRECTIVES [Dir]

c. Respects the patient's freedom

1. LINGUISTIC DEFERENCE [LD]
2. [Potentially non-PCC] TOUCHING WITHOUT ASKING [TW]

Figure 3.1 Face-PCC analytical categories

I also present a category 'potentially non-PCC' that refers to opposite examples that potentially fail to accomplish PCC. I consider the non-PCC elements as 'potential', as there are several assumptions that can arise within the particular situation. The non-PCC acts can occur when the doctors prioritise their professional agenda rather than identifying the patient's face needs, which could be rooted in the doctor's authority to be in charge of treatment. Non-PCC acts can also occur as a result of missing an opportunity to achieve PCC, due to various causes such as the provision of more complicated explanations and patients' strong initiatives. However, all aspects of PCC are strongly related to the relationship between the doctor and patient over time. This means that, when the participants' mutual face needs are supported overall, PCC acts may be achieved even though out of context, individual formulations may appear to be non-PCC. Therefore, non-PCC potential is estimated in context but not with absolute certainty.

For the identification of the categories, some borderline cases were observed and considered with respect to the interactive exchanges. Particularly, the subcategories of empathy and shared decision-making have some overlaps, and they required careful evaluations in order to minimise the possible overlapping of categories; therefore, the classification and borderline cases will be discussed further. The categorisation of the data was the key to analysing the discourse and finding the characteristics of the participants' speech acts.

The analytical categories are explained and illustrated in detail below, including excerpts of the transcripts and explanations of how the examples fit the category. The superordinate terms are highlighted in bold italics, the subordinate terms in italics and sub-subordinate categories in capital letters so that these can be distinguished from the rest of the descriptions. The number in the square brackets next to each example corresponds with the case number.

I. Attends to Patient's Positive Face

The first superordinate category includes physicians' statements and responses that attend to the patient's positive face (the desire to be accepted, praised and appreciated for an affirmative self-image). As one of the features of the data, the physicians visit their patients' homes fortnightly, and in some cases, they have had an established relationship for years. The professionals' linguistic forms would change depending on the current level of the relationship with the patient, and their friendliness needs to be considered in the whole discourse, as far as this may be retrieved from the context. Three main PCC categories are subordinated to ***Attending Patient's Positive Face***: (a) *Identifies issues that the patient wishes to address*, (b) *Actively listens to the patient* and (c) *Displays empathy and acceptance*. Opposite examples that potentially undermine accomplishing PCC are also included for each category.

I.a. Identifies issues that the patient wishes to address

The skills involve two subcategories: INITIAL GENERAL REMARKS and GRADUALLY MOVES FROM OPEN TO CLOSED QUESTIONS. First, the physicians' initial remarks at the beginning of the consultation, which are commonly made following greetings, include general enquiries (e.g. *'How are you doing?'*) or follow-up enquiries (*'How's the back pain?'*). These can also be statements to introduce tasks (*'Let me take your body temperature'*). Initial general remarks express interest in the patient's state of health or progress with medication, demonstrating that the professional notices the patient's condition. Because attending to positive face can be used as 'an accelerator of interactions' in general (Brown & Levinson, 1987: 103), the initial general enquiries in the initiation stage has the function of enhancing the patient's positive face. Examples of INITIAL GENERAL REMARKS include:

'How are you doing?'
'It's very cold today, isn't it.'
'Isn't there any change?'

The follow-up questions are often formulated as semi-open questions (starting with *'How's...?'*) and are followed by further closed questions, which gradually narrow down the questioning. This questioning sequence is categorised separately under *I.b Actively listens to the patient*, as it is more oriented towards identifying the patient's specific health problem and is likely to be a safe strategy by which the physician stresses his or her willingness to find out more about the patient and thus satisfies the patient's face need (i.e. to be accepted). Examples of GRADUALLY MOVES FROM OPEN TO CLOSED QUESTIONS include:

'Have you struggled with constipation for a long time, right? [...] How long have you had that? Since what age...?'

'Is there any change for your stomach? [...] Does it still feel painful? You now don't take diuretic medication, right? [...] How about your leg swelling?'

The opposite strategy, SEQUENCE OF CLOSED QUESTIONS AT THE BEGINNING includes examples where the physician immediately starts to ask the patients or their families a closed question sequence without general enquiries, or uses the same approach to ask the patient's family about the patient, such as in:

'The other day, you had blood in your urine again, hadn't you? Two days? Did it stop? Didn't you have stomach-ache or something like that? [...] Wasn't that much as last time? Not much? Just once?'

'It looks like there is not any change with her (speaking to the patient's family in the patient's presence while looking at a notebook that has

records by the patient's carer). It looks like she eats well, and her bowel movement is good. Okay. Haven't you fallen, right? (to the patient)'

These sequences are potentially non-PCC.

I.b. Actively listens to the patient

This category includes REPETITION, PARAPHRASING AND INTERPRETATION, which considers the physician's repetitions, paraphrasing and interpretation of the patient's statements that help to elicit information and/or the patient's perspectives. This appears similar to the previous category above, GRADUALLY MOVES FROM OPEN TO CLOSED QUESTIONS. However, this category does not necessarily take the form of questioning but includes repetitions or paraphrasing of a word or phrase, which satisfies the patient's desire to be listened to. This aspect, which relates to encouragement, eliciting more information, ideas, expectations and feelings from the patient, is also a prerequisite to *I.c Displays empathy and acceptance* and *II.a Works towards shared decision-making*. The studies reviewed in Chapter 1 showed that listening to the patient without interrupting is well accepted by patients, and one of the specific listening skills includes the physicians' strategic use of repetitions, pauses and clarifications. This category, therefore, is particularly concerned with the attentiveness of listening and related techniques that may encourage the patient to express their views and stories further. However, I consider this process of generating information at this phase as an example of active listening and have not double coded as empathic skills or shared decision-making in the analysis. Examples of repetition, paraphrasing and interpretation include:

'Yes'; 'I see'; 'You cannot sleep... right.' (repetition)

'Right. Your back tends to bend, right?' (paraphrasing)

'You haven't been good. So, it's not something specific, but feeling like... (it's not good) about lying down itself.' (paraphrasing)

'You feel easier to go up the stairs rather than coming down, don't you?' (interpretation)

'Oh, really! It's like this? (using gestures)'

The opposite category, INTERRUPTION, includes examples where the physician interrupts the patient's or patient's family's talk before they finish. These are potentially non-PCC formulations, as in:

'You said something different about it last time... (interrupts the patient talking about an argument with family). Then you had an argument... (interrupts the patient's statement and appears to close down the topic) ... I see. You argued about it.'

'Last time, you said that you had some pain on your ankle... (interrupts the patient, "Yes, it has been...") It's been painful? ... (interrupts the patient, "It was okay for two weeks...") Has it returned? Same here, right?'

I.c. Displays empathy and acceptance

First, UNDERSTANDING AND APPRECIATION OF THE PATIENT'S FEELINGS refers to the physician's obvious acknowledgement of the patient's expression of concerns, fears, feelings and thoughts. This involves not simply the identification of what the patient said but also the appreciation of the patient's underlying emotions and views and extends to validity and willingness to support. Examples of UNDERSTANDING AND APPRECIATION OF THE PATIENT'S FEELINGS include:

'When you feel pain, you really don't have to stand or hesitate to take medication.' (understanding)

'I guess you are feeling motivated about it... I hope you start to take a walk when you want to.' (appreciation)

'I think you've been doing very well. [...] You don't have to work too much for it.' (appreciation)

'That must be painful and a shock...' (understanding)

Second, EXPRESSIONS OF POSITIVE REGARD include praise and reassurance as a form of acceptance. The examples illustrate specifically how the physician picks up (or misses) a potential opportunity to demonstrate positive regard, such as in:

'Right. You think like that... It's hard for your body, but I think it's great that you take such positive views.' (acceptance)

'You're fine. Good. Your husband looks fine, too.' (assurance)

'You have a very good posture when sitting down ... I think the centre of your body looks very stable. It's good.' (reassurance)

'Stay healthy during the winter.' (encouragement)

'It's very important for you to eat well and gain physical strength.'

'It's (your feet) become much better... Ah, that's good.' (encouragement)

Lastly, SILENCE AS EMPATHIC ANTICIPATION is classified as an empathic behaviour here, rather than as part of active listening, as the examples from the data frequently demonstrate silence (much longer than a pause) to be eliciting the patient's emotions. The data will furthermore illustrate that the nurses' utterances can be significant in expressing encouragement and empathy to the patient before the physician's first response. Examples of SILENCE AS EMPATHIC ANTICIPATION include:

Silence that elicits the patient's feelings:

Patient:	*My joints are worn out, and they don't work... I cannot sit down.*
Doctor:	*Yes...*
	(5.0)
Patient:	*I don't know how to say...*
Doctor:	*Yes...*
	(4.0)
Patient:	*I get irritated about myself because I cannot move...*
Doctor:	*Ah...*
	(4.0)
Patient:	*Only my hands move, like this.*
Doctor:	*Yes, yes...*
	(8.0)
Patient:	*When I lie down, my back hurts.*
Doctor:	*Ah, I see.*
	(3.0)
Patient:	*All around my back is painful, and I feel like punching someone to get them to do something about it.*
Doctor:	*I see. ((sigh))*

The opposite category, BEING JUDGEMENTAL, refers to potential examples in which the physician appears to blame the patient for not doing appropriately. These are potentially non-PCC formulations, as in:

> '*You went to the day-care centre, didn't you? [...] You didn't go. You should go in that case. [...] Not that day, but the following day. You'd better go in such case.*'

II. Attends to Patient's Negative Face

The second superordinate category involves physicians' statements and responses that attend to the patient's negative face (i.e. the desire to be independent, be unimpeded and autonomous). This is at 'the heart of respect behaviour' (Brown & Levinson, 1987: 129) and occurs particularly in situations in which the empowerment and balancing of power is required, such as in shared understanding and/or a shared decision-making, because it performs the function of minimising the imposition and potential pressure on the patient. Three main PCC categories are subordinated to *Attending to the patient's negative face*: (a) *Works towards shared decision-making*, (b) *Leaves space for the patient* and (c) *Respects the patient's freedom.*

The category of *Works towards shared decision-making* is highly cultural- and/or context-dependant; this could significantly vary depending on a culture. In this study, most of the corpus within the process of shared decision-making turned out that the data involved a high degree of negative politeness strategies rather than positive politeness strategies in the consultations. Thus, it is classified under *Attends to Patient's Negative Face*. The data also show numerous variations in the uses of polite expressions that show the distance and power in the participants' relationships and, thereby, attend to the patient's negative face wants. The use of polite form is often investigated at the sentence level rather than at the discourse level; in this study, I considered forms of LINGUISTIC DEFERENCE that express respect to the patient in specific contexts but do not cover the use of the Japanese honorifics (polite form) in detail. Instead, I primarily focus on the linguistic behaviours chosen to accomplish a particular aspect of PCC in the discourse. Opposite examples that potentially undermine accomplishing the PCC features are also included for each category.

II.a. Works towards shared decision-making

The category SHARING UNDERSTANDING concerns the physician's attempts to reach a collaborative understanding of the patient's problems. This process, then, aims to reach a shared agreement in the decision-making process rather than one-way information-giving from the professional, which often included face-threat mitigation. In order to allow the patient to understand the process of shared decision-making, the doctor would be expected to share their own ideas as well as elicit the patients' through facilitating skills. Examples of SHARING UNDERSTANDING include:

Planning medication:

Doctor: *I wonder about the tablet you take for your bowel movement...*
Patient: *That's right. I want to take more.*
Doctor: *You want to take extra, right? Is your stool soft?*
Patient: *Yes, it is, sometimes. But it depends.*
Doctor: *I see. If you take extra, stool may become too soft....*
Patient: *Ah...*
[...]
Patient: *It's been difficult. I would like to try other medication to improve my bowel movement. Wouldn't they work at all?*
Doctor: *I think other treatment would work. We could try.*

The skills to involve the patient in the process of shared decision-making also concern the next category, SHARING THINKING. The doctors may share their thought processes on treatment plans and alternatives and give information. These processes largely involve the listening techniques seen above, such as using repetition and summarising, as well as expressing understanding the patient's situations. The professionals also combine those listening and empathic skills in this phase of shared decision-making. I considered this entire process as one instance of this category and therefore did not double code it as listening or empathic skills in this analysis. Examples of SHARING THINKING include:

> *'Basically, you don't need to take tablets for your cystitis. As your previous doctor said, having water will help to cure it [...] If you had taken medicine indecisively, well, have you heard "resistant bacteria"? [...] for the future, the medicine might become ineffective, so it's normally said that you shouldn't take antibiotics excessively [...] Shall we do just water next time? [...] Without taking antibiotics, shall we try?'*

> *'It is fine to stop taking the tablets, but if you stop it abruptly, some people start feeling pain. Gradually, it should be weakened [...] Let's have weaker one (30 seconds of silence while checking the patient's record) Considering your liver condition, I think the current one is weak enough for you [...] We can stop it this time, and let's see how it goes [...] I think, even though we stop it now, it should be no problem in this situation.'*

The process of shared decision-making is generally followed by the third subcategory, OFFERING SUGGESTIONS, where the physician encourages the patient to contribute their ideas. This is an important step to get the patient involved in the next decision-making process. Particularly, the presence of family members can affect the patient's decision-making because it reveals whether the patient is involved in the essential process. The physician often uses the forms, *'Let's...'* or *'Shall we...'* across these three subcategories, which highlight the cooperativeness of the physician's action towards the patient. Examples of OFFERING SUGGESTIONS include:

> *'Another issue to discuss is whether we increase the number of the tablets for your bowel movement [...] I know that you would like to have more (the same tablets) [...] But it might not help that much [...] What shall we do? Would you like to have more?'*

> *'I'm going to prescribe the same medicine today [...] How's the condition of your stomach? [...] If the condition is stable, I think we can reduce the amount of digestive [...] You can continue to take it, or you can reduce or stop it. What would you like?'*

The opposite category, NO SHARED DISCUSSION, concerns examples where the physician's explanation potentially appears dominant and the patient's ideas are hardly asked for, even though the patient or the patient's family state their disagreement explicitly or implicitly. These are potentially non-PCC formulations, as in:

<u>Missed opportunity of a shared discussion:</u>

Patient: *This medicine... my stool was too soft every day, so I stopped taking it just for the mornings.*

[...]

Doctor:	*Do you know what this medicine is? [...] I cannot say there is no relationship between this medicine and stool. But I cannot say that they're absolutely related to each other. If there are any risks of stopping the medicine, it would become harder when you urinate, and at the worst, urine would be accumulated without coming out. It's called 'urinary obstruction.'*

II.b. Leaves space for the patient

The category, OPEN QUESTIONS THAT OCCUR THROUGHOUT THE SESSION, may occur throughout the consultations, particularly after greeting and initiation. The reason why open questions are considered both as forms by which the physician may address negative face as well as positive face (in the very first category, INITIAL GENERAL REMARKS) is that the function of, and the information generated by, an open-ended question may be different depending on the stage of the consultation. While open questions in the initiation stage are used to express socially expected opening remarks, an open question at a later stage gives space to the patient to consider their options or express their views or interests. Examples of OPEN QUESTIONS THAT OCCUR THROUGHOUT THE SESSION include:

<u>Open question during the physical exam:</u>

Doctor:	*Let me take your body temperature. The weather is getting better, isn't it?*
Patient:	*Yes.*
Doctor:	*You can see the cherry blossoms soon.*
Patient:	*I'm not interested in that.*
Doctor:	*Oh really. What are... well, what do you enjoy?*

Second, CHECKING FOR UNDERSTANDING involves the physician's skills of providing feedback to the patient, at any stage of the consultation, regarding what they have heard and understood. This may include checking whether the patient understands the professional's thoughts, before proceeding to the next chunk of information, ensuring that the patient is comfortable with the plan and allowing them to ask for any corrections or clarification. This behaviour eventually ensures understanding on both sides: the doctor understands the patient, and the patient understands the doctor. Examples of CHECKING FOR UNDERSTANDING include:

<u>Repetition of important points by the doctor:</u>

Doctor:	*Today, I'll give you painkiller as usual, compress (against legs), and medicine for the stomach that helps improve bacteria getting better. We'll reduce this from six to three tablets.*
Patient:	*Ah, did I take it as many as six?*
Doctor:	*Yes.*

<u>Restatement of information by the patient's family and doctor:</u>

Doctor:	*You need the same tablets, right?*
Family:	*And compress.*
Doctor:	*Yes. Compress, and ointment.*
Family:	*Yes.*
Doctor:	*I will give you compress and ointment.*

The opposite category, DIRECTIVES, shows examples where the information appears to be delivered as a one-sided speech and is too prescriptive. These are potentially non-PCC formulations, as in:

<u>Potentially prescriptive advice:</u>

Doctor:	*Did your previous doctor tell you that you need to finish taking it for seven consecutive days, once you start taking it? [...] If you take antibiotics, it should be taken for a week properly. If you don't take it, it should be none. Either zero or seven days.*
Patient:	*I was careless.*

II.c. Respects the patient's freedom

This last subcategory considers LINGUISTIC DEFERENCE, including conventional indirectness, thanks and apologies. Such deference does not merely respect the patient's freedom but also reduces potential risks of misunderstandings. The relevant expressions are often used during the physical examination because the doctor physically touches the patient's body. Culturally, touching in a medical context may strike the patient as discomforting or disturbing (Crezee & Asano, 2016). Because even an everyday word can be ambiguous in the medical consultation, the physician attempts to use various expressions ranging from indirect or more descriptive. Examples of LINGUISTIC DEFERENCE include:

<u>Explanation before injection</u>

Doctor:	*I am going to inject you now, around here. The disinfectant will feel a bit cold. You may feel a slight pinch.*
Patient:	*It (being said) will make me feel more pain.*
Doctor:	*I'll be careful... ((laugh))*

<u>Expressions of apologies when leaving in a hurry:</u>

Doctor:	*Would it be possible for me to go to the next patient's place. I'm sorry... The tea and chocolate were delicious.*
Patient:	*Yes, yes. I'm sorry for forcing you to stay.*
Doctor:	*Thank you very much.*
Patient:	*No, no, I've been forcible...*
Doctor:	*Next time, see you again.*
Patient:	*Yes. I appreciate that you always listen to me.*
Doctor:	*Excuse me.*

The opposite category could potentially concern examples of unmitigated orders or similar acts. As far as physical touch is concerned in this study's context, the category TOUCHING WITHOUT ASKING can be placed here. This includes touching the patient without asking for permission or appropriate verbal introduction, resulting in the patient's discomfort. This is implicit to potentially non-PCC formulations, as in:

Touching without asking
Doctor: *How's swelling on your leg? Hasn't it changed?*
(5.0)
Patient: *It's painful when it's touched!*

3.16 Conclusions

I have applied mixed methods, taking advantanges of the qualitative designs and tools to capture naturally occuring conversations in the authentic consultations. This approach follows both deductive and inductive reasoning in that it starts with existing theories but it is then modified on the basis of observations and data. Initially, I formulated the key sequence patterns for generalisations on the basis of existing theories of PCC and Face. However, my fieldnotes and one-to-one interviews with the physician participants contributed further important insights for the interpretation of the naturally occuring interactions in the consultations. One problem could be that, while the literature describes how important non-verbal behaviours are in clinical practice, video recordings were not available during the fieldwork, and I was not able to record non-verbal behaviours accurately. My interpretation largely relies on the details of the participant's talk, tone of voice, pauses, silences, noise, the literature, textbooks, materials, and the fieldnotes describing room layout, sitting positions, noticeable gestures the participants made, the patient's background, lifestyles and talks conducted outside of the consultations.

Another issue is the possible interference of the researcher, as the existing literature warns (Epstein *et al.*, 2005; Gold, 1958; Potter, 2002). My impression was that the participants hardly deviated from their usual styles of interacting with each other, because I carried out multiple observations sitting in for one patient without recordings for many cases. This gave me the confidence that the participants' behaviours were seldom affected by recordings, particularly in clinical consultations where their tasks were fixed. The English translations were wholly checked by the professional translator as exaplined in Section 3.13, and I made sure that these translations are truthful representations of the original meaning and added functional words only when they were needed for the reader to understand. In the following chapters, clear examples are presented and illustrated, starting with the doctors' attentive listening skills in Face-PCC categories emerging from the analysis.

Note

(1) This is a similar distribution to the one provided in the government's official report on patient demographics in Japan (Cabinet Office Government of Japan, 2018).

4 Listening to Patients and Identifying Issues

This chapter will now illustrate the physician patient-centred communication (PCC) communicative acts emerged from the analysis, focusing on their listening techniques and identifying issues that the patient wishes to address (the full details of the instances from the Face-PCC analysis are presented in Appendix 9.3). Extracts from the analysed consultations are selected to present the specific linguistic instantiations of the represented Face-PCC categories, *Identifies issues that the patient wishes to address* (I.a) and *Actively listens to the patient* (I.b). The extracts are presented in frequency order of the subcategories rather than the timeline of the consultation so that the reader can first see the common sequence patterns of the physician expressions.

4.1 Doctor's Facilitative Responses

Elicitation through the doctor's questioning techniques is seen as one of the foundation skills of PCC. Facilitating responses includes statements made by the physician that encourage the patient's expressions about such aspects as their subjective experience of the illness or disease, their ideas, expectations, needs, symptoms and functioning. Starting with greetings (e.g. '*Good morning. How are you today?*'), the doctor's facilitating responses can consist of broad opening, open-ended questions (e.g. '*Tell me about the pain, will you?*'), listening while encouraging, echoing and interpreting (e.g. '*Uh, uh*', '*Go on*', '*Do you think you are stressed out?*'), use of silence, indicating understanding (e.g. '*I see*', '*Right*'). In such exchanges, the patients' knowledge, and subjective experiences (e.g. what is wrong with them, what might be causing it, etc.), as well as their psychological functioning, can be generally explored; Stewart *et al.* (2014) claim that PCC encompasses weaving back and forth between these two perspectives. Although these exchanges occur simultaneously with non-verbal facilitation, the type of verbal responses and their (in)frequency can be analysed in detail by considering their cultural characteristics.

4.2 Evidence of Active Listening (I.b)

REPETITION, PARAPHRASING AND INTERPRETATION (I.b.1) in *Actively listens to the patient* were the frequent PCC communicative acts in the data and identified in 20 cases. They were explicitly displayed in clarifying the patient's history, especially for more focused questioning in the initial phase of the consultation. In particular, the physician listening skills were notably seen when they spoke to older patients with hearing impairment. The opposite category as potentially non-PCC, INTERRUPTION (I.b.2), was identified in three cases for Consultations A (patients attending on their own) and one for Consultations B (patients attending with their families and/or friend or neighbour).

The following extracts show how doctors applied the PCC acts to encourage the patient's narratives. Participant roles are abbreviated as follows: physician (D), resident physician (RD), nurse (N), assistant (A), patient (P), patient's family (PF: e.g. patient's son: PF-S) or care manager[1] (CM).

4.2.1 REPETITION, PARAPHRASING AND INTERPRETATION (I.b.1)

Extract 1 is one of the clearest examples of speaking to older patients with a hearing impairment. The 94-year-old male patient was in a wheelchair and lived in a nursing apartment (residential building having individual rooms and live-in caregivers). The doctor was standing while facing the patient directly, and two resident physicians were standing one at each side. They spoke to him slowly and distinctly. Repeating a single word that the patient said (Line 9), the doctor further slowed down and stressed the word clearly (Lines 13, 19, 21). This gave the patient a chance to focus attention to an event, which led to facilitating the patient talking about his friend at length for three minutes.

(1) Case 2, A: Repeating a single word

		((D and RD check vital signs))
7	D	**Do you go out?** ((asking the P's life world)) お出かけはしてますか↑
8	P	**Eh?** はい↑
9	D	**<<u>Outside</u>.> [Going out,** ((stressing a single word)) <そと.> 外出 [は,
10	P	**[Aha. Well, I went to Ginza** (**downtown**) **the day before yesterday.** [ええ (.) ええ. あのね, おとといは銀座まで行ってきました.
11	D	**Ah, <u>I see</u>!** あ, <u>そうですか</u> : :
12	P	**By taxi.** タクシーで.

13 D **By taxi. [Well…**
タクシーで. えっと : : [なに,
14 P **[I said to my friend, "let's drink in Ginza".**
[友達と銀座で一杯やろうって.
15 D **Oh, really!**
お : : そうですか : :
16 RD **Oh…**
お : :
17 D **<Your friend…>?**
<友達> っていうのは : :
18 P **Yes. It's funny. He's three years older than me.**
ええ (.) それがね, 面白いんですよ. 僕より三つ上なんですよ.
19 D **Three years older.**
三つ上.
20 P **Though I say a "friend", he was my senior colleague when I was working. He's 97...**
友達って言ってもね, 会社にいたときの先輩になるんですけどね.
97ですから : :
21 D **97.**
97ですね.
22 P **Anyway…**
we went to a nice nostalgic (.) [grilled chicken] restaurant.
[…]
それで : : 昔なつかしい (.) 焼き鳥屋がありまして.

The doctor and resident physicians added slight exaggerated tones of voice for their facilitative comments *'Oh, really!'* (Lines 11, 15, 16), which signalled their interest in his story. The repetition of a single word from the patient's phrases encouraged the patient to continue with his narrative.

In other cases, there was a combination of such repetition and non-verbal gestures. In Extract 2, for example, the patient's feet were swollen, and she explained that she had suffered from swelling of the feet since she was young. The participants repeated the word *'like this'* (Line 64) with a prolonged sound of voice, and the doctor repeated the same sound while swinging his arms and echoing, as follows:

(2) Case 9, A: Combining with gestures

57 P **Then, I used to have an injection every day…**
それで注射 (.) 毎日毎日して,
58 D **Ah, you had an injection,**
((repetition))
あ (.) 注射して,
59 P **I had. I dropped by a [clinic, when I commuted.**
してたの. [お医者さん (.) 通るから, 行ってる間はね.
60 D **[Ah, I see. Right, right.**

((facilitative comment))
[ああ (.) そうですか. うん (.) うん.

61 P **I wasn't able to wear shoes like these at that time.**
そのとき, こんな靴なんて, 履けなかったもんね.

62 D **Oh really!**
ああ本当ですか.

63 P **Yes. Now it's fine, (2.0) but, here,**
my legs had become <like this.>
((prolongs the sound and swings the arm))
そ. 今はさ, 全然 (2.0) ここ, 〈こ : : んな (.)〉 なっちゃってたもん.

64 D **((laugh)) Here, <like this>?**
((D imitates the same sound and move))
hhh ここ (.) 〈こう : : なってね.〉

65 P **Yes, yes, <like this.>**
((P and D repeat the same move))
そうそう. 〈こう : : ね.〉

66 D **Ah, I see…**
ええ : : そうですか : :

67 P **A long time ago, they said "eat cooked barley"**
昔はね, 麦のご飯食べろって言われてた.

The prolonged sound '*like this*' (Lines 63, 64) and the repetitions of the gesture elaborate how her legs were badly swollen in those days. These exchanges encouraged the patient to continue with her narrative about her experience (Line 67).

Facilitative comments and interpretation were often used to respond to the patient's implicit expressions of feelings. For example, in Extract 3, the patient, who received palliative care at home, stated her pessimistic views '*There's nothing I can do*' (Line 39). She is a terminal patient suffering from myeloma and has had inflammatory reactions and bone pain.

(3) Case 10, A: Neutral interpretation

34 D **Are the symptoms around here still the same?**
Does it still feel painful?
ここら辺の症状は, 相変わらずですか :↑苦しい感じ↑

35 P **They haven't changed. It'll continue… unless I grow taller.**
相変わらず. それはもうね (.) 背が伸びない限りは.

36 D **Right, right.**
うん (.) うん.

37 P **You know, (4.0) I feel like I'm getting shorter…**
なかなか (4.0) 少しづつ縮んじゃうのが[ね : :

38 D **Right. Your back tends to [bend, right?**
[うん. 腰がね. [曲がってしまってね =

39 P **[Yes. There's nothing I can do.**
[うん. それはしょうがない. うん (.) うん.

40 D **You feel pressure on your stomach, right?**
= お腹が圧迫されてね.

41	P	**Yes, that's what the disease is, <u>you know</u>.** うん. そういう病気だから<u>ね</u>.

The doctor describes how she would feel about her pain. The reason this example is categorised as active listening rather than expressions of empathy is that the skills used in this extract are neutral comments such as *'yes'*, *'right'*, *'…right?'* and the doctor adds interpretation of the patient's last phrase (Lines 36, 38, 40). This does not go further to assess or show understanding but seems neutral and simply facilitative.

The three examples above have portrayed how the doctors took several minutes of time to encourage the patients to keep talking, using verbal and non-verbal facilitative neutral words.

The use of repetition was more common in Consultations B. In Extract 4, the patient living with her daughter's family spends most of the day in bed. For the first half of the consultation, the professionals and the patient's family discussed the patient's lung condition and asked the patient afterwards how she felt. The doctor called her name and spoke clearly so that the patient could pay attention to what the doctor was saying.

(4) Case 15, B: Repetition and clarification

95	D	**(P's name) how are you feeling now?** ((open question)) (P's name) 具合はどうですか (.) 今.
96	P	**Fine, I suppose.** 別に, 大丈夫です.
97	D	**Fine, you suppose?** 別に大丈夫.
98	P	**Yes.** はい.
99	D	**Your daughter said that you've had loose bowels…** うん (.) お腹が緩いって : : お嬢さんが言ってるけど : .
100	P	**Um, something like loose bowels…** Um : なんかね, 便が緩い : .
101	D	**Loose.** ((repetition of a single word)) 緩い.
102	P	**I also had stomach pain… but I have recovered from it.** お腹も痛かったけどね : : もう治った.
103	D	**You've recovered. How's your appetite?** もう治った. 食欲はどうですか↑
104	P	**Ah, I have an appetite.** ああ (.) あります.
105	D	**You have it, too. // You're fine.** 食欲もある. // 大丈夫.
106	P	**// Yes, yes.** // はい (.) はい.

Repetition is used in a similar way as in the previous extracts (Lines 97, 101, 103, 105); however, this example includes an element of clarification, which could also lead to SEQUENCE OF CLOSED QUESTIONS AT THE BEGINNING (I.a.3), and potentially be non-PCC. However, the doctor refers to the worries of the patient's daughter (Line 99), and he intends to check it out. After the patient mentioned that his condition had improved, the doctor asked another question on her appetite, which he tactfully extended to further enquiries. Otherwise, the patient would have had less chance to speak to the professionals. Her responses, overall, are very short, providing only brief clarification. This example is closer to the boundary between active listening and closed-ended questioning.

Similarly, the following Extract 5 also shows how the doctor uses repetition and paraphrasing for in-depth clarification. The distinct aspect of this extract is that all the participants can understand what the patient has said and what is going on by the doctor's verbal responses. Through one-to-one interview with the doctor, I found out that this was an intentional strategy. The patient has Parkinson's disease and lives with her daughter. She was also residing at a short-stay nursing home for a couple of days a week. The family worried that she often vomited at the nursing home. The patient tended to speak very fast and close her eyes; these phenomena are both characteristics of the disease. The doctor sat facing the patient directly and repeated her utterance almost every time. The family and nurse were present in the same room and understood what she said.

(5) Case 18, B: Repeating almost all the utterances

75	D	**Were you unwell almost every day?** 毎日のように気分が悪くて↑
76	P	**Yes, I vomited.** ええ. もどしたの.
77	D	**Were you feeling ill and then vomited?** ((paraphrasing)) なんか (.) 気持ち悪くてオェっていう感じだったんですか↑
78	P	**Yes.** はい.
79	D	**Oh, dear... Was it just once or several times?** あら本当 : : 一回だけもどしたのかしら (.) 何回か,
80	P	**It seemed like my stomach was overwhelmed...** 胃がびっくりしたみたい : :
81	D	**It seemed like your stomach was overwhelmed.** ((repetition)) **Just once? Several times...?** ((clarification)) びっくりしたみたい. 一回だけ ですか 何回か : :
82	P	**I vomited twice.** 2回くらいもどした.
83	D	**You vomited twice. Hmm...** **Did you feel a little better after vomiting?**

2回くらいもどした. Hmm :. もどしたあとはちょっとスッキリしましたか?
84 P **Yes- Hmm, not that much.**
うん- そう ::: でもないですね.
85 D **Not that much. Umm. How about at home?**
そうでもなくて :: Umm :: おうちではどうです↑
86 P **I vomited at home as well.**
おうちでももどしましたね.
87 D **You did. Did it happen during the daytime?**
もどしました. Umm :: それは (.) 昼間ですか↑
88 P **Daytime.**
昼間.
89 D **Daytime.**
昼間に.
90 P **Yes.**
ええ.
91 D **Hmm… Morning or afternoon?**
Hmm :: 午前中, 午後↑
92 P **Well, late afternoon, I think…**
えっと, 夕方だったかな ::
93 D **Late afternoon. I see.**
Did it happen after you ate snacks or something?
夕方くらいに ああ :: そうですか. なんかおやつかなんか食べたあとですか?
94 P **Yes…**
そう :: ね.

For almost every utterance, the doctor repeated the last few words that the patient said and then asked what he wanted to ask. The doctor also checked her recall, asking for the time when things happened. The doctor, physician participant D3, explained that he applied several skills more consciously now to mitigate the patient's anxieties, and another doctor D4 also recollected her perception of why she could not perform well when simply speaking to patients (the full transcripts of the interviews with the original text are provided in Appendix 9.4):

> I have changed how I respond while listening to the patient's story, especially whether to let something pass without comment, whether to remain silent, when to add empathetic phrases, and so on, but these changes were only in minor or insignificant details. These are certain skills to build a better relationship with patients, in order to draw them towards us [health professionals] emotionally, or to remove as much anxiety as possible. [D3: Paragraph 5]
> 話を聞きながらどういう風に返答するか、流すか、沈黙をとるかとか、どのタイミングで共感的なフレーズを入れてみるかとかそういうところは変わってきたと思いますけど、枝葉が変わったという感じです。より効果的に関係性を作るために、患者さんの気持ちをこちら側に誘導するため、もしくは不安を取り除くためにです。

He also responded that he consciously tries to check the patient's words by repeating and clarifying the meaning, so as to avoid a potentially paternalistic style of consultation:

> If you're not repeating or paraphrasing, it's easy to often misread someone's intentions. Japanese people especially tend to smile and sidestep things. The man we first met today is hard of hearing, and probably he didn't hear what I said. But I think he thought that it would be rude if he asked me to repeat what was said in that situation, so he just nodded and said 'yes, yes.' I can check if I have misheard what the person has said, but it's difficult to check about what I have said, unless I consciously confirm it with the patient. Especially when the patient is smiling and saying 'yes, yes', I carefully think about what that 'yes' means. If you do not listen attentively and dig for more information or confirm the patient's words, or ask opinions with an appropriate introduction, the interaction can easily take a structure like 'Please do whatever you want, doctor.' [D3: Paragraph 12]
> リピートもパラフレーズもしないと、意図を読み取り違えていることもしばしばあるので、特に日本人はわからないとニコニコ誤魔化す。　今日最初にお話された、男性の方なんかは、あの方も耳が遠くて、おそらく言ってた言葉は聞こえてなかったと思うんです。でも、あの状況で、聞き返したりとかしたら、失礼かもなと思って、ああ、はい、はい、って形で頷いたと思うんです。　向こうが言ったことは聞き違えがないかの確認ができるけど、こちらが言ったことは伝わってるかどうかは意識しないと、笑ってハイハイと言われるとね、何のハイかなと思うんです。意識して少し掘り下げたりとか聞き直したりとか、枕詞を入れた上で意見をお聞きするとかしないと「先生のいいようにしてください」とそういう風になりやすくなるのは構造上あると思います。

This statement refers to an important aspect underpinning the hierarchical relationship between the patient and doctor in Japan. Fujisaki (1997) explains that Japanese patients tend to place their emotional trust in doctors, summed up in the words: 'I am a lay person and do not have medical knowledge. Please do whatever you think is best'. Fujisaki states that this does not mean that the patients underestimate their own judgement, but rather that this is a strategic act to emotionally elicit the optimal support from the doctor. In other words, passive attitudes in Japanese patients could be interpreted as an act to save the doctor's face by expecting a better outcome. Some professionals reconcile with this cultural tendency. However, Fujisaki (1997) states that such traditional, hierarchical doctor–patient relationship can collapse as the practice of in-home medical consultations expands. This is because some doctors are wary of falling into potential paternalistic styles as D3 explained and consciously attempt to create equal balance by involving the patient.

Below, the last extract in REPETITION, PARAPHRASING AND INTERPRETATION (I.b.1) is an example of when the doctor makes sounds (non-verbal) and uses tone of voice to show his attentiveness. The patient lived with her husband and was staying at a short-stay nursing home for a couple of days a week. Her husband explained to the doctor that she was recently treated a little violently at the nursing home. The doctor responded by uttering a sound that appears to convey his understanding of how hard this must be for her.

(6) Case 19, B: Sound and the tone of voice

24	PF	**It seemed like she was treated a little violently when she went to the bathroom.** あの (.) トイレの時に, ちょっと乱暴に扱われたみたいなの.
25	D	**When she went to the bathroom. [Really.** ああ : : おトイレの時ですか (.) [ほんとに.]
26	PF	**[Yes.]** [うん.]
27	D	**Roughly, like this?** (4.0) グッとみたいな感じ↑
28	P	**They sat me down on the toilet seat with <a bump.>** 便座にね, < ど : : ん > と座らせたの.
29	D	**Ah… a bump!** ((making a louder sound)) あ : : どんって.
30	P	**Yes.** そう.
31	D	**Aah… (3.0) that must have been painful and a shock…** ああ : : (3.0) 痛いし, ちょっとショックなのもあるし : :
32	P	**Yes…** そうね…
33	PF	**So, on Sunday, she said her leg hurts.** それで日曜日にね, 足が痛いって.

By making sounds accompanying *'Roughly'*, *'bump', 'Aah…'* (Lines 27, 29, 31), the doctor expressed understanding for the seriousness of the event the patient experienced. Although the patient's responses were simply *'yes'*, these assisted the patient's husband to represent and tell the story for her. The phrase *'that must be painful and a shock'* is an expression of understanding and empathy; these combinations of listening and empathy were commonly applied in most of the consultations.

Overall, the six extracts above have portrayed how the doctor's facilitative responses functioned as encouragement for their patients' personal narratives, and some of them indicated how the narrative could be restricted by the doctor's request for clarification, especially when they have more participants in the consultation. The particular skills used for speaking to older patients with hearing impairments have also been illustrated. The professionals would stand or sit facing the patient and spoke slowly and distinctly. There also is an indication for the correlation between the frequency of the PCC acts and the topic initiation and enquiry phase. Repetition was applied not only to facilitate the talk but also to ensure that all the participants in the room could understand what the patient said. The tone and speed of voice were also part of the skills demonstrated by the professionals.

4.3 Evidence of Identifies Issues That the Patient Wishes to Address (I.a)

Performing open-ended questioning at the beginning of the consultations was uncommon in the data, particularly in the consultations with the patients on their own. INITIAL GENERAL REMARKS (I.a.1) were relatively common when the family was present (in Consultations B), whereas these remarks were fewer when the patients were on their own (in Consultations A). SEQUENCES OF CLOSED QUESTIONS AT THE BEGINNING (I.a.3) as potentially non-PCC were more frequent, which is further discussed in Section 4.4. The professionals tended to initiate close-ended questioning that followed up a problem from the previous consultations while checking vital signs, which was the major cause of the infrequency of the feature GRADUALLY MOVES FROM OPEN TO CLOSED QUESTIONS (I.a.2). However, the professionals made more non-medical conversations when the patient's family was present; this happened because the physician often used semi-open questioning styles and did not focus on the patient's problems immediately, as the family often provided a clarification of the problem on their own initiative. Thus, GRADUALLY MOVES FROM OPEN TO CLOSED QUESTIONS (I.a.2) was more commonly practised in Consultations B.

INITIAL GENERAL REMARKS (I.a.1) were often accompanied by POSITIVE REGARD (I.c.2) in Consultations A, as in Extracts 7 and 8:

4.3.1 INITIAL GENERAL REMARKS (I.a.1)

(7) Case 9, A: General enquiry

1	D	**Is there any change?** 何か変わったことありましたか↑
2	P	**Nothing.** ないです.
3	D	**You're fine. Good. Your husband looks fine, too.** 大丈夫ですか. よかった (.) ご主人もまあそんなに, 変わらなそう : :

(8) Case 14, A: General enquiry and positive regard

1	D	**(P's name) how are you?** 調子はいかがですか↑
2	P	**Good.** いいです.
3	D	**Good. (3.0) You drank tea well just now, didn't you?** いいですか (3.0) 今の, お茶の, 飲み具合も, 良かったですね.
4	P	**Ah. Did I?** ああそうですか.

In most consultations analysed, the patient's initial reply was frequently a short word such as *'good'*, *'fine'* or *'nothing (has changed)'*. The doctor's responses were often followed by an echo of the patient's word and encouragements such as *'that's good'*.

As shown in Extract 7, it was common for the doctors to express that they also had an interest in knowing how the patient's family had been (Line 3). For Extract 8, since the patient had a gastrostomy tube through his belly, the doctor told the patient, *'You drank tea well just now, didn't you?'* (Line 3) to acknowledge his stable condition.

Extracts 9, 10 and 11 illustrate examples of INITIAL GENERAL REMARKS in Consultations B. In Extract 9, as soon as the doctor and assistant started checking vital signs of the patient at the beginning, the wife of the patient's brother checked the patient's foot, which had developed swelling due to thrombus. Establishing a common ground by making initial remarks about the cold weather (Lines 1, 3), the doctor immediately asked a semi-open question (Line 4) to the family member.

(9) Case 21, B: Topic of weather

		((D and A start checking vital signs))
1	D	**Your hands are cold today, too.** 今日も (.) 手冷えますね.
2	P	**Yes.** ね.
3	D	**On a chilly day like today, our hands get cold.** 今日みたいに寒い日は. 手がね. 冷たい.
4	D	**How is it?** ((asks PF who's checking the patient's foot)) どうですか↑ : :
5	PF	**She doesn't seem in pain at all.** 全然痛がらないんです.

Extract 10 reverses the process: the doctor established a common ground with the family first, showing that the professionals had noticed the patient's stable condition (Lines 1, 3), and then asked the patient a follow-up question (Line 5).

(10) Case 22, B: General enquiries to both family and patient

1	D	**It looks like there is not any change with her, right?** ((asks PF, reading notes that PF has recorded on P's status)) 変わりない : : [ような感じですかね.
2	PF	**There's no change.** [変わりないですね : : はい.
3	D	**It looks like she [eats] well and** **her [bowel movement] seems good. Okay.** よく [食べて] るし, [お通じも] 出てます. オッケーです.
4	PF	**[Yes.] [Yes.]** [はい.] [はい.]

5	D	**Haven't you fallen?** ((asks P)) 転ばなかった[です↑
6	P	**Ah, no I haven't.** [あ, 大丈夫です.
7	D	**Okay. £ That's very good £.** ((encouragement)) オッケーですね : : £はい (.) とてもいいです£.

In Extract 11, the doctor asked an open question after she finished checking and recording the patient's vital signs (Line 11), not during the check as happened in other extracts above.

(11) Case 26, B: Open question after pause

1	D	**Shall we measure your blood pressure and so on?** ((D and A check vital signs)) じゃ血圧とか測りましょうかね. [...]
11	D	**How are you?** どうですか (.) 調子の方は.
12	P	**Bad.** わるい.
13	D	**Bad.** ((repetition)) わるい. (2.0)
14	P	**I think I am going to die from this.** これで死ぬんだろうなって気がする.
15	D	**You think you are going to die from this.** ((repetition)) これで死ぬんだろうなって気がする.

The doctor recognised that the patient often stated sadness and frustration about his debilitating long-term condition. It appears that the doctor took the time to listen to and deal with the patient's emotions after realising the seriousness of the patient's condition in Extract 11 (Lines 13, 15). This dialogue led them to discuss how the patient was feeling frustrated at himself.

4.3.2 GRADUALLY MOVES FROM OPEN TO CLOSED QUESTIONS (I.a.2)

Although the open-ended questions were not used frequently at the beginning, the professionals appeared sociable in the presence of the patient's family, which helped them to apply semi-open enquiries and perform GRADUALLY MOVES FROM OPEN TO CLOSED QUESTIONS (I.a.2). Extracts 12 and 13 show how open and semi-open questions provide the patient with time to recall and answer at some length and how the physicians take the opportunity to provide encouragement or further clarification.

(12) Case 17, B: Open and semi-open questions

1 N **Then, let me measure your body temperature first.**
はい (.)じゃ : : 先にちょっとお熱を測りますよ : .
2 P **Okay.**
((N checks vital signs))
はい.
(9.0)
3 D **How are you doing?**
((open question))
調子はどうですか↑
4 P **Um, not much has changed…**
う : : ん : あんまり変わらないんだよな : : .
5 D **Um… How's your back?**
((semi-open question))
Um : 腰の塩梅はどうです↑
6 P **Well, only for my back, it [doesn't hurt anymore.**
あのね, そこだけはね, [痛くなくなった.
7 D **[I see. Ah, £ that's good £. I see.**
((encouragement))
[ええ,] あ, £それは良かった£. そうですか.

In this Extract 12, it is notable that the doctor's second enquiry sheds light on the positive aspect of the recovery. The patient initially answered in a lower tone of voice '*not much has changed…*' (Line 4) after the doctor's initial enquiry '*How are you doing?*'. The patient then stated in a brighter tone of voice, '*only for my back, it doesn't hurt anymore*' (Line 6) after the doctor's second enquiry, a semi-open question, '*How's your back?*' (Line 5). The doctor expressed encouragement, as the patient had recently taken medication for the back pain (Line 7).

Slight differences can be seen in Extract 13, which illustrates the way of establishing common ground '*It's very cold today, isn't it?*' (Line 1) at the beginning, echoing (Line 5) and a clarification of a problem that had occurred previously to smoothly move from open to closed questions (Lines 3, 7, 9).

(13) Case 19, B: Multiple means to move from open to closed questions

1 D **It's very cold today, isn't it?**
((topic of weather))
今日は (.) だいぶ寒くなりましたね : :
2 PF **Yes, yes.**
うんうん.
3 D **How are you?**
((open question))
調子 (.) どうですか↑

4 P **It's okay.**
調子はふつうです.

5 D **Okay?**
ふつうですか↑

6 P **Yes.**
はい.

7 D **Hmm... When I visited you before,**
Hmm : この前は- あの- 伺った時は =

8 P **Yes.**
はい.

9 D **you said that at night you hadn't had scary dreams lately, [but, how's it going currently?**
((a follow-up question))
=ちょっと怖い夢(.)最近見なくなったわって(.)仰ってた[けど,最近どうかしらね.

10 P **[I haven't.** ((**laugh**))
[ええ. £見ません£ hh

11 D **You haven't? Ah, good. £ I see £.**
見ません? あよかった. £そうですか£.

The key feature for the doctor's exploration at the beginning of the consultations was performing open-ended questioning, although it was identified in small number of instances. The professionals tended to immediately follow-up the problem from the previous consultations. However, in Consultations B, they appeared making non-medical statements and more laughs, which helped them to apply broad (semi-open) enquiries. Multiple combinations of the skills such as general enquiries, positive regard, reassurance and encouragement were often applied.

4.4 Potentially Non-PCC Elements

SEQUENCE OF CLOSED QUESTIONS AT THE BEGINNING (I.a.3) was coded as the opposite category of the PCC indications and was commonly practised. Extract 14 is an example of the sequence without general enquiries at the beginning of the consultation. The full transcript (see also Appendix 9.5) includes the exchanges of a closed question sequence that lasted for four minutes, in which the doctor clarified the patient's history on her blood urine, symptoms and actions that she had taken. Although she did not seem reluctant to answer all the questions, her answers were very short.

(14) Case 4, A: Closed questioning to clarify the history (example of I.a.3)

3 D **The other day, you had blood in your urine again, didn't you?**
この間 (.) 血尿がまた出てしまったんですよね↑

4 P **For two days.**
二日間.

5 D **Two days?**
二日間↑
6 P **After I took (the tablet),**
飲んだら,
7 D **Did it stop?**
うん (.) 止まりました↑
[…]
((many closed questions to clarify the patient's history))
45 D **Right. Have you been urinating more frequently than before or do you have pain when you urinate?**
Any symptoms like that?
((multiple questions))
[…]うん. おしっこが今までよりも (.) 頻繁に出るとか,
おしっこする時に痛いとか (.) そういうのはなかったですか↑
46 P **It['s] not painful, but it is frequent.**
痛くはないで[す.] でも頻繁ですね.
[…]
51 D **Well, it's the same as normal, which [was] frequent to begin with, and it hasn't changed, has it?**
ま(.)いつもとは変わらない(.)もともと頻繁に(.)[あって,]
変わらないということですね↑
52 P **[(hh)] Yes.**
はい.

This technique can be seen as assisting the patient in recollecting the past events and define the problem; however, rather than providing assistance or guidance, this appears to be more directive with less exploration and more medical perspectives.

Similarly, Extract 15 shows how rigidly the course of closed-ended questioning was operated. At the beginning, the doctor immediately gave the result of a blood test, which was followed by reassurance (Line 1). The doctor then only asked closed questions relating to the patient's appetite and bowel movement (Line 6). When the patient missed a question, the nurse intervened and navigated to answer the missed question (Line 11).

(15) Case 12, A: Course of closed-ended questions (example of I.a.3)

1 D **The test result last time was very good.**
Your urine has no problem at all.
この間の検査結果は (.) とてもいいですね.
おしっこの方 (.) 全く問題がないです.
2 N **You are fine. Rest easy.**
((D and N check vital signs))
大丈夫です. 安心してくださいね.
[…]
6 D **Do you eat meals?**
お食事は食べて[ます↑
7 N **36 degrees.**
[36度です.]

8	D	**36 degrees exactly.** ((writes down)) 36度ちょうど.
9	N	**Doctor asked, how about meals?** お食事はどうですかって.
10	P	**Yes.** はい
11	N	**Doctor asked you if you are able to eat?** お食事は食べれてるって (.) 今, 先生が聞きました.
12	P	**Yes, I do.** はい. 食べてる.

Some examples are difficult to label as non-PCC, especially when the professionals' acts and/or tone of voice seemed to address the patient's problems seriously. The following Extract 16 includes task-oriented statements only. The patient was supposed to be hospitalised again two weeks after this consultation. The professionals immediately asked if the date was confirmed (Line 2) and gave a prescription straight after that (Line 7). The exchange might appear directive; however, the overall atmosphere is relatively relaxed – the participants were sitting in a dining room, and the patient was preparing tea to offer her guests.

(16) Case 13, B: Task-oriented initiation (example of I.a.3)

1	N	**Excuse me.** ((D and N check vital signs)) じゃ : : すみません. (12.0)
2	D	**(You don't know) when you'll go into hospital next, do you?** 今度の入院日とかは (.) まだ,
3	P	**I think it would probably be early April…** あ, たぶん4月の上旬 [じゃないかと思うんですけど : .
4	D	**Early April.** [上旬ですね.
5	N	**Haven't you heard anything (from the hospital)?** まだ連絡がない [んですか↑
6	P	**Yes, yes. I expect to get a call from the hospital soon, but it's up to them …** [はい. はい. あ (.) また連絡が入って来ると, 期待してるん ですけど, 病院次第なもので : :
7	D	**I see. Today, I am going to prescribe the same medicine for one month.** そうですよね : : いつも通り今日は, 一ヶ月分 [お出ししておいて,
8	P	**Yes, please.** [はい. はい. お願いします.

In cases where the doctor only asked closed questions at the beginning, the initial phase of the consultation tended to be occupied with history-taking or administrative tasks as shown above. This could also be associated with doctors' interruptions; although INTERRUPTION were identified in few instances, they seemed to occur as a result of clarification seeking.

Extract 17 is one of the obvious examples of INTERRUPTION (I.b.2). The doctor's first statement overlapped with the resident physician's (Line 2), and the next statements interrupted the patient telling her story (Lines 4, 6, 10).

(17) Case 3, A: Interrupting the patient's story

1	RD	**Let me take your body temperature and blood pressure.//** 体温とか血圧とか (.) 測ります//ね.
2	D	**//Well… <u>last time</u>, you said that you had some pain on your ankle…** //あの: : 足首前も痛いって仰ってたけれど : :
3	P	**Yes, it's been [painful all this time.** そうなんです. ずっと [痛いって,
4	D	**[It's been painful all this time?** [ず : : っと痛かった↑
5	P	**It wasn't sore for about [two weeks], but…** 痛くないときがあった [んですけど2週間] くらい.
6	D	**It [wasn't sore] for a short period. Has it returned?** [痛くないときがあった.] またぶりかえした↑
7	P	**Yes.** ええ.
8	D	**Is it in the same place?** 同じ場所ですか↑
9	P	**It's not painful if I keep it <u>like this</u>.** **When I start [walking…** <u>こうやって</u>れば痛くないんですよ. で (.) 歩き出す[と : :
10	D	**[Right.** [うん.

Although the technique of closed questions is not necessarily considered as a disadvantage, it seems to noticeably influence the flow of information exchange and the patient's narrative because there is little space and time for all the participants to listen and think.

4.5 Conclusions

Physician facilitation, REPETITION, PARAPHRASING AND INTERPRETATION (I.b.1) were explicit, and clear examples were identified in almost all the consultations. The communicative acts are grouped and summarised in Table 4.1. A significant effect of repeating the patient's words is that all the participants in the consultation can understand what the patient has said and what is going on by the doctor's verbal responses. The one-to-one interview with the doctor revealed that he does so intentionally so

Table 4.1 Summary of the communicative acts in *Listening to Patients and Identifying Issues*

Category of Face-PCC	Features
I.a. Identifies issues that the patient wishes to address	• INITIAL GENERAL REMARKS were particularly used in Consultations B where the families were present and included: ▪ General enquiries to both the family and the patient ▪ Open question after a pause ▪ Topic of weather • GRADUALLY MOVE FROM OPEN TO CLOSED QUESTIONS included: ▪ Open and semi-open questions ▪ Multiple means to move from open to closed questions • [Potentially non-PCC] SEQUENCE OF CLOSED QUESTIONS AT THE BEGINNING was the most common demonstration of non-PCC and included: ▪ Closed questioning to clarify the history ▪ Course of closed-ended questions ▪ Task-oriented initiation
I.b. Actively listens to the patient	• REPETITION, PARAPHRASING AND INTERPRETATION were commonly identified in almost all the consultations, and particularly used for speaking to older patients with hearing impairment. These included: ▪ Repeating a single word ▪ Combining with gestures ▪ Neutral interpretation ▪ Repetition and clarification ▪ Repeating almost all the utterances ▪ Sound and the tone of voice • [Potentially non-PCC] INTERRUPTION included: ▪ Interrupting the patient's story

as to avoid adopting a potentially paternalistic style of consultation. Another distinct feature at the beginning of the consultations was that SEQUENCES OF CLOSED QUESTIONS AT THE BEGINNING, which are potentially non-PCC, were commonly seen, mostly in Consultations A for the patients attending on their own. The professionals tended to initiate close-ended questioning to follow-up a problem with those patients, and conversely, the doctors often made more INITIAL GENERAL REMARKS when family members were present.

Note

(1) The professional role, care manager, has overall responsibility for planning care for older adults in the local government, and thus, more professionals can intervene in the patient's care. When several other plans are involved in the care of the patient (such as visiting nurses in addition to the physician home visit), the doctor brings the discussion back to the patient's care manager, who will then adjust the care plans with the professionals involved. In some cases, care managers attend the medical consultations and speak to the doctor on behalf of the patient or family.

5 Empathy and Acceptance

Empathy, as one of the key elements of patient-centred communication (PCC), is understood as the doctor's engagement beyond the simple eliciting of experiences and perspectives. Empathy refers to doctors' elicitation and responses that acknowledge patients' emotions and feelings, whether they are expressed explicitly or implicitly. Doctors' empathy, therefore, specifically aim at picking up patients' expressions of emotions and feelings, as opposed to merely acknowledging fact-based events of their illness experiences.

In healthcare contexts, clinical empathy has been defined as 'a cognitive attribute that involves understanding a patient's suffering and concerns combined with an ability to communicate this understanding and an intention to help' (Hojat *et al.*, 2015: 12). The term 'clinical empathy' is commonly used in medical practice (Brugel *et al.*, 2015). In demonstrating PCC, it is assumed that the doctor attempts to understand the patient's psychosocial context by attending to the feelings regarding beliefs, spiritual issues, financial aspects, social roles, struggle and life crisis and taking an individual focus. Particularly in the interactions between physicians and older patients in their continuous care, PCC can also include topics related to the broader life context and end of life care.

Lawrence *et al.* (2004) summarise the concept of empathy defined in psychology, noting that two principal dimensions of empathy exist: *cognitive empathy* and *emotional empathy*. Emotional empathy can be further divided into two dimensions, *parallel* and *reactive* emotional empathy, the latter of which can be manifested in sympathy. It is important to distinguish empathy from sympathy for someone's suffering. Northouse and Northouse (1997: 24) describe sympathy as 'concern, sorrow or pity shown by an individual for another individual. It is the expression of one's own feelings about another person's predicament and the urge to alleviate his or her suffering'. This often refers to compassion, as it means 'suffering with'. Goetz *et al.* (2010: 351) define compassion as 'the feeling that arises in witnessing another's suffering and that motivates a subsequent desire to help'. In Hojat's (2007) publication, *Empathy in Patient Care*, he shows a graphic presentation showing the relative contribution of cognition and emotion in empathy, sympathy and compassion, and how they overlap (Hojat, 2007: 11). In the graphic presentation, empathy is positioned in the area of *cognition* rather than *emotion*, and conversely, sympathy is positioned in the area of *emotion* rather than *cognition*. There is a small area of the overlap between empathy and sympathy, where compassion resides. All these components have the capacity for better person-centred communication between patients and professionals.

The interactional sequence involves answering questions, agreeing with assertions, demonstrating understanding and showing feelings. Wynn and Wynn (2006) note that when empathy is expressed, the patient must receive it by responding appropriately to the professionals' prior utterances. With particular attention to its verbal aspects, empathy-relevant expressive features in medical consultations are conceptualised in terms of 'Empathic Speech Acts' (Pounds, 2011, 2018; Pounds & De Pablos-Ortega, 2016), which are specifically concerned with eliciting and acknowledging the patients' emotions and feelings and conveying positive regard and support to the patients. Pounds' framework, 'Empathic Speech Acts' (2011) distinguishes doctors' potential empathic verbal expressions between (a) eliciting the patient's feeling and views and (b) responding to the patient's cues, in each respective speech function. Responding to the patient's cues extends it to expressing 'acceptance' including 'unconditional positive regard (or praise)' and 'neutral support'; these dimensions require more than facilitation as understood in the context of an interview, requiring doctors to engage both cognitively and behaviourally.

In Japan, the concept of empathy is recognised as a Western notion, and the differences of the nuances of 'sympathy' and 'empathy' are rarely revealed. Expressions of empathy are often tied to posture, gesture, reflection and the provision of clarifications, as outlined in the Objective Structured Clinical Examination (OSCE) guidelines referring to 'empathic communication skills' (Common Achievement Tests Organization, 2020). Although Japanese literature has recently begun to discuss this theme of clinical empathy, several textbooks address the fact that medical staff often face strong emotions from patients, such as anger or sadness. In these cases, expressing empathy is defined as understanding the sequence of events that stimulates these feelings in patients and responding with understanding (Suzuki & Abe, 2011: 11). Son *et al.* (2018) measured Japanese medical students' willingness to show empathic behaviours, using a self-assessed scale for measuring empathy, the Jefferson Scale of Empathy for students (Hojat *et al.*, 2001, 2002; Kataoka *et al.*, 2009). The result shows that the students' empathic behaviours were more correlated with 'perspective taking', which is a cognitive component and is distinguished from the compassionate care that is an integral part of sympathy. Indicating understanding verbally and non-verbally seems to have a substantial role in the medical students' behaviours. Pounds *et al.* (2018) developed an empathy-specific medical admissions interview station, probing applicants' empathic communicative performance at medical school and fitting in the Multiple Mini Interview (MMI) format. It is hoped that additional measure of empathic communication can be used in health educational and professional settings and adapted to support student and staff selection in other professional contexts. The underlying context – the difficulty of empathic and compassionate care – has long been addressed in the Western context (Jeffrey, 2016; Scott *et al.*, 2008; Soto-Rubio & Sinclair, 2018), since traditionally, medical students used to be taught to be detached and uninvolved with patients' strong emotions. However, unempathic responses can create difficulties in doctor–patient relationship, and realisation of empathy – perhaps particularly verbal expressions – is needed in performing PCC.

5.1 Evidence of Empathy and Acceptance (I.c)

The findings of the Face-PCC communicative acts show that EXPRESSIONS OF POSITIVE REGARD (I.c.2) were the most frequent expressions and evenly seen in both sets of Consultations A and B. For UNDERSTANDING AND APPRECIATION OF THE PATIENT'S FEELINGS (I.c.1), on the other hand, the category showed a difference: more sequence patterns of empathy in Consultations A (patients attending on their own), and only four patterns in Consultations B (patients attending with their families and/or friend or neighbour). SILENCE AS EMPATHIC ANTICIPATION (I.c.3) was observed in three cases in Consultations B, but was infrequent in Consultations A. The opposite category as potentially non-PCC, BEING JUDGEMENTAL (I.c.4) was also infrequent; two cases were identified in Consultations A. The extracts are presented in frequency order of the subcategories so that the reader can first see the common sequence patterns of the expressions.

Below, Extract 18 shows an example of how the doctor acknowledged the patient's desire to walk and expressed positive regard. The patient had a pacemaker and used to suffer from low back pain due to a compression fracture. The doctor had suggested that she should start rehabilitation walking (the full transcript of this case is included in Appendix 9.5).

5.1.1 EXPRESSIONS OF POSITIVE REGARD (I.c.2)

(18) Case 4, A: Combination with giving some space

87	D	**Okay, we talked about rehabilitation last time.** **Did you talk to your care manager about wanting to try it?** はい. この間(.)リハビリの(.)お話：をしたら, リハビリちょっとやってみようかなってお話が, ケアマネさんに ありました↑
88	P	**Yes.** はい.
89	D	**It seems you're feeling a bit more motivated about it.** ね, 少し (.) やる気になったのかしら.

90	P	**I think I want to try walking.** 歩いてみようかと.
		[...]
98	P	**But it's not ideal when it's so cold...** でもあん：まり寒い時はね：：
99	D	**Yes, that's right.** うん, そうですね.
100	P	**Once it gets warmer outside. Um, we talked about that, so,** ちょっとあったかくなったらね. あの (.) 話しておきましたので,
101	D	**Right, then, around when the cherry blossoms bloom,** あ, そうですか (.) じゃ (.) 桜が咲いたらとか,
102	P	**hhh** ((laugh))
103	D	**Right? Around when the weather gets nicer.** ね, いいお天気になってきたら (.) とかね.
104	P	**Yes.** そうですね.
105	D	**Once the weather gets nice enough that you want to take a stroll, it would be great if you could start around then. Yes.** お散歩したくなってきたらね. 始められるといいですね (.) うんうん.

The doctor's initiation *'It seems you're feeling a bit more motivated...'* (Line 89) acknowledged the patient's desire to walk. She also showed her understanding of the difficulty of walking in the winter (Lines 101, 103), visualising the patient walking in the nice weather a few months later. This example is a combination of positive and negative face. The last phrase (Line 105) attends to the patient's negative face, which implies that there is no need to do the rehabilitation right away and gives space and time to the patient.

Extract 19 is an example of offering reassurance. The patient lived with her bedridden husband and looked after him. Before starting this initial enquiry, the doctor and nurse had checked her husband's condition and returned to the room where the patient was sitting. Starting with a semi-open question regarding her condition, the doctor offered encouragement and a reassurance that her husband looked fine. The initial enquiries also included asking about her husband as well.

(19) Case 9, A: Reassurance by including family

1	D	**Has there been any change?** 何か変わったことありましたか↑
2	P	**Nothing.** ないです.
3	D	**You're fine? That's good.** **Your husband looks the same as usual, too.** 大丈夫ですか. よかった(.)ご主人もまあそんなに, 変わらなそう：.

4 P **Yes.**
はい.
5 D **Well, just now, he said that he'd experienced strong stomach pain. Had you noticed?**
なんかさきほど(.)すごくおなか痛い時あったって, 仰ってましたけど,
そんなことありました↑
6 P (3.0) ((silent))
7 D **It wasn't really a big deal?**
そんなに大騒ぎするほどじゃなかった↑
(4.0)
8 P **No.**
はい.
9 D **Ah, today we have brought an injection.**
Shall we do it later, after taking your blood pressure and doing an examination?
そうだ, 注射のお薬も(.)今日持ってきているので,
血圧とか診察のあとに注射もしましょうね.
10 P **Yes.**
はい.

In most of the data in Consultations B, it was commonly seen that the professionals showed their interest in the patient's family members. The doctor checked up on the patient's husband, which would ideally be of comfort (Lines 3, 5, 7), as he understood that she had been looking after him on her own. The doctor's last utterance also follows the inclusive form *'Shall we do...'* (Line 9), when indicating what they would do in the consultation.

Extract 20 also shows that the patient with Parkinson's disease was pessimistic about going outside and viewing the scenery, because she tended to close her eyes due to the characteristics of the disease. The doctor spent a few minutes with her practising opening her eyes, while praising her for doing well. The patient's responses were short, but her laughter became louder towards the end of the extract. This is an outstanding example of the doctor's willingness to assist the patient and illustrates the practice of combining the attentive skills.

(20) Case 18, B: Praising for doing well

37 P **I cannot help closing my eyes (2.0)**
even though the cherry blossoms are out...
桜が (.) 咲いても：, (2.0) 目をつぶっちゃって,
38 D **You cannot help closing your eyes?**
目をつぶっちゃって,
39 P **Yes.**
はい.
40 D **Umm, open your eyes nice and slowly. Yes, yes, yes.**
It's very good that you open your eyes nice and slowly.
((encouragement))

		Umm ゆっくりゆっくり開けるとね, そうです, そうです, そうです, ゆっくりゆっくり (.) 開けていくとね, いいと思うんですよね.
41	P	**I tend to shut my eyes firmly…** かたく閉ざしちゃうんですよね (.) 目が.
42	D	**You tend to close your eyes so tight,** ((repetition)) **so it's good that you open your eyes nice and slowly.** **The longer you close your eyes,** **the more your eyes tend to stick together.** **Yes. It looks very good when you open eyes slowly.** ((praise)) どうしてもかたくね, 力が入りやすくなるので, ゆっくりゆっくり目を開けるといいと思うんですよね. 長く閉じてるとね, 目が少しくっつきがちになっちゃうので. そうですね. ゆっくり開けるととってもいいですね.
43	P	**£ I see £.** ((laugh)) £ そうですね £ hh
44	D	**I can see your best smile of the day.** ((praise)) 今日一番いい (.) 素敵な笑顔が見られた.
45	P	**hhh** ((laugh))

The previous three extracts, i.e. Extracts 1, 2 and 3, are examples of giving reassurance and encouragement that were most commonly seen in the category of empathy. These skills were associated with allowing some time and also including topics raised by family members. Extract 3 also demonstrates that the doctor was willing to help the patient to practise opening her eyelids and overtly displayed a combination of encouragement and praise (Lines 40, 42, 44).

In Extract 21, the doctor listened to a terminal patient suffering from myeloma. I remember the setting of this consultation: jazz music flowed through the room, the tone of the patient's voice was cheerful, and she offered tea and confectionary, as if nothing was wrong with her. In fact, I later learnt that this patient often called the doctor to talk about her sadness and spiritual pain, and in the consultation, she commented on how her own personality may be the cause of her disease. The doctor tried to turn the patient's pessimism into a positive outlook by adopting a neutral stance, neither agreeing nor disagreeing with her views (Lines 257, 259), whereas the patient thought that the situation was all her fault.

(21) Case 10, A: Positive regard and withdrawing judgement

256	P	**Well ah… as the cause of my disease,** **my (impatient) personality was probably my ruin.** あの : : まあ : : 病気の原因 (.) そういう性格[が, あの : : 災いしたのかもしれない.
257	D	**Right… You think like that.** うん : : そういう風に思われてるんですね.

258 P **Yes, I [do.]**
うん, 思っちゃう[のね : .]
259 D **[You think] so. I don't think so though.** ((laugh))
[思っちゃう.] そんなことはないですけどね. hhh
260 P **Really?** ((laugh))
If it isn't the case, that would be… Yes, I feel like <u>that</u>.
hhh £そうかな. £そうだと<u>あれ</u>なんだけどね (.) そんな感じでね.
261 D **Yes.**
うん.
262 P **I think I should have a more easy-going attitude.**
ちょっともっともっとのんきに構えなきゃと思って.
263 D **Right. I see. You're going to change your way of thinking.**
うんうん. なるほど. 考え方を変えていかないと.
264 P **Yes, yes. I tend to overthink things.**
I get absorbed in my illness.
そう (.) うん (.) 考えすぎのところがあるんでね,
こう病気の中にのめりこんじゃう 自分がね.
[…]
267 D **It can't be helped to some extent.**
You cannot move because of the disease.
ある程度は仕方ないですよね.
だって病気があるから動けなくなってしまったわけだから.
268 P **Not much. It's a shame to be controlled by a disease, right?**
But, all the physical challenges are because of the disease…
あんまりね(.)その, 病気に支配されるっていうのもね, あの : :
情けない話で(.) でもまあ, いろんな不自由になる原因っていう
のは(.)
病気なわけだから.
269 D **Yes. That' right.**
うん : : そうですよね.
[…]
282 D **It's hard for your body… but,**
I think it's great that you take such positive views.
お体は辛いけれど : : 前向きにね,
考えられてらっしゃるところはね, 素敵なところですね.

The patient's self-blame and vagueness were frequent in her utterances (Lines 256, 264, 268). Although the doctor maintained neutrality, she also expressed a disagreement '*You think like that. I don't think so though*' (Line 259), implying that blaming herself was wrong. While rejecting the patient's view could potentially be unemphatic, the rejection of her self-blame appears EXPRESSIONS OF POSITIVE REGARD, as the patient responded with a vague sense of relief about being told so (Line 260), which shows that the doctor's denial was not a threat but rather, a comfort that mitigated any implied judgement. The vague expression '*like that*' (Line 260) was frequent in this patient's utterances. The doctor's skills in listening to the patient's spiritual pain also required accepting her views (Lines 267, 282). In the end, the doctor showed encouragement for her efforts in trying to think positively.

5.1.2 UNDERSTANDING AND APPRECIATION OF THE PATIENT'S FEELINGS (I.c.1)

Showing understanding for the patient's feelings and views tended to be followed by visualising positive outcomes. In Extract 22, the doctor acknowledged the patient's struggle in looking after his bedridden wife and his anxiety about it. The patient had previously broken his legs and was hospitalised for two months until recently. Meanwhile, the wife's condition was getting worse, and the challenge for the patient included the question of how to care for his wife while caring for himself. Considering the circumstances, the doctor responded by showing his understanding.

(22) Case 11, A: Combining understanding and positive imagination

95	D	**There are many positive sides of walking, right?** いい部分も沢山ありますでしょ↑ 歩くと.
96	P	**Yes.** (2.0) **I feel that I should walk more.** ええ. (2.0) 自分ではね, 歩いた方がいいなっていう,
97	D	**I see. That's great.** ((encouragement)) そうですね. 素晴らしいですね.
		[...]
107	D	**Caring for your wife occupies a lot of your mind, doesn't it?** ((understanding)) 奥様のケアっていうのは (.) 今頭の中にかなりあるでしょう↑
108	P	**Yes, yes... it does. It's almost only about care for her.** ええ, ええ : : あります. もうほとんど, 彼女のケアだけですから.
109	D	**So, I think what you've done (walking) is very useful. You've followed the right direction, one that is reasonable for you.** ((positive regard)) だから, そういうのには(.)すごく役立つと思います. 今の方向性はすごく, 大変理に適ってるし,
110	P	**Yes. I am thinking the same way.** うん (.) それは自分でも思ってますからね.
111	D	**Excellent.** ((positive regard)) 素晴らしいです.
112	P	**hhh** ((laugh))

The doctor's display of understanding that the patient's situation must have been difficult gave the patient an opportunity to explain his thoughts about caring for his wife (Line 107). The doctor's supportive statements were followed by acceptance that justified his walking activity (Lines 95, 109) and encouraged him (Lines 97, 111). These additional displays of empathy – for example, the extra acknowledgement for the patient who looked after his spouse at home – was one of the salient aspects in this context.

Below, Extract 23 shows the doctor addressing the patient's depression by rephrasing his feelings. The patient suffered from a debilitating long-term condition, drug allergies, as well as pain in his back and legs. Thus, he could not take appropriate medication or engage in physical therapy. He told the doctor that he was feeling frustrated about how painful always being in bed was. The doctor sat at his bedside and spoke to him in a lower tone of voice; these verbal and non-verbal behaviours demonstrated appreciation for the patient's feelings.

(23) Case 26, B: Tuning the tone of voice to the patient's depression

113	P	**I feel, like, listless…** なんか::気だるいっていうか,
114	D	**You feel listless… or you don't feel refreshed.** ((paraphrasing)) 気だるいっていうかね::スッキリしない.
115	P	**I don't feel refreshed.** スッキリしない.
116	D	**We'll have to work on it at a lazy pace.** ((laugh)) ボチボチやっていくしかないですね hh (4.0)
117	P	**Well, I've been [unwell for a long time…** もうなんかこんな具合悪く[なって, 長いこと,
118	D	[Yes. Yes.] [うん. うん.]
119	P	**Even at the university hospital, they said they cannot help me.** 大学病院でもしょうがねえなあって. (5.0)
120	D	**Shall we do a blood test again next week, when I come next time?** **Well, for your heart and liver,** **the previous test results weren't that bad.** またでも来週ちょっと採血してみましょうか.次回来る時. あの, 心臓とか肝臓とか,今までの採血もそんな悪くないんですけど, […]
133	P	**Well, nothing can help.** **I hope I can slowly slide down to death.** まあしょうがないよね.このままずるずる, 死ねればいいけど.
134	D	**You hope? You think so?** いいけど↑そう思う↑
135	P	**I cannot die easily, can I?** なかなか死ねないんだよな. (2.0)
136	D	**We shall work on it slowly.** ちょっとだらだらね, やっていきましょうね.

While listening, the doctor occasionally laughed a little or used a cheerful tone of voice (Lines 116, 136), which could soften the formality of the consultation and introduce a more caring tone. This appeared to encourage the patient to talk about the fact that even the hospital couldn't discover what was wrong with him. The stressed words 'lazy pace' (Line

116) and 'slowly' (Line 136) appear to emphasise how things may be done, albeit at a slower pace for him.

I often observed situations where an older patient mentioned *'I want to die'*. This was also discussed in one-to-one interviews with the physician participants. According to physician D1, this is one of the most common difficulties that all physicians face in the settings with older adults, in terms of how to respond to feelings of hopelessness that the patient can have.

> When I see older patients, I often hear the phrase 'I want to die' and think how I should respond to the statement, because you cannot show no reaction. If you do not say anything and leave without changing your facial expression, you are a robot. If you are told 'I want to die, doctor', you will be moved because you are a human, and the one who has to think of a response is the medical worker. This is not taught in medical school. This matter tests our powers of humanity and communication skills. [D1: Paragraph 12]
> 高齢者の方を見ていると、よく死にたいという言葉を聞くので、そこにどう答えていくかという。それを言われた時に、レスポンスゼロというわけにはいかないので。もし何も言わないで、何も表情一つ変えずに帰ってしまったら、ロボットですよね。人間だから絶対、死にたいと言われたら心を動かされるし、何か答えなきゃと思うのが医療従事者。そこは学校で教わらないこと。そこは自分の人間力とか、コミュニケーション力が問われるとは思います。

Supportive comments were also often seen when the patients expressed their fear, which was occasionally followed by giving advice. However, the doctor would not miss the patient's cue and would also express appreciation for their feelings, especially for patients in difficult situations. In Extract 24, the patient had numbness in his legs and was receiving rehabilitation. Encouraging him to continue to do the exercises, the doctor effectively used his knowledge that it was important for him to maintain the current situation rather than seek immediate improvement.

(24) Case 27, B: Picking up the patient's fear

103	D	**Oh, you do it (walking) on rainy days as well?** あ (.) 雨降った時もやってるんですね↑
104	P	**Yes.** ええ.
105	D	**That's great!** 素晴らしいですね.
		[...]
108	P	**It's fine when I go up, but I feel scared when I go down.** 上がる時はいいんだけど下がるときが怖くてね.
109	D	**Ah...** あ : :

110	P	**When the floors are wet when it rains…** なんかね (.) 雨降っててあの濡れてると,
111	D	**Ah… I see.** あ :: そうですよね :. […]
		[…]
115	D	**For example, you can go up the stairs, and use the elevator to go down, perhaps.** あの (.) 例えばね, 階段で上がって, エレベーターで降りるとかでも(.)いいかもしんないですね.
116	P	**Ah… just go up to the top, and,** あ :: 上がるだけ上がって,
117	D	**Yes.** **You feel much easier when going up the stairs, don't you?** うん (.) 上がりのほうが安心じゃないですか↑
118	P	**Somehow, yes.** はい. なんだかね.
119	D	**Right.** うん.
120	P	**I am scared.** 怖いんです.
121	D	**I see. Yes. I understand.** そうですね. うん (.) わかります.
122	P	**I know there is nothing to be scared of.** 怖いこと (.) ないんだけどね.

Many elements can be observed in this extract: the doctor acknowledging the patient's practice on rainy days (Lines 103, 105), showing awareness of the patient's fear (Lines 109, 111, 117) and giving a suggestion about using an elevator to go down (Line 115), as well as making constant facilitative comments. The patient appeared pleased to be understood and receptive to the brief advice in the end.

Overall, the previous extracts, i.e. Extracts 22, 23 and 24, were examples of UNDERSTANDING AND APPRECIATION OF THE PATIENT'S FEELINGS (I.c.1) and also included frequent expressions of acceptance, which demonstrate the professionals' sensitivity towards the difficulties of the patients. These communicative acts were accomplished through tone of voice and picking up cues. The array of empathic skills is achieved from listening to the patient's narrative carefully and attending to the emotional needs.

5.1.3 SILENCE AS EMPATHIC ANTICIPATION (I.c.3)

As the unique feature of this category SILENCE AS EMPATHIC ANTICIPATION (I.c.3), silence was often utilised when the patient was assumed to be difficult to handle for the professionals. Three cases were identified for this category, and all three of the patients were male.

In Extract 25, the patient seemed to be suffering from a sleeping problem and wished to have extra tablets that would make him sleep better.

The doctor explained at length that the tablets must not be increased as it would make him drowsier thereby increasing the risk of falling and rejected the patient's request (Line 101). However, the patient held out for the tablets and seemed positive about managing the drowsiness that would result from taking extra tablets (Line 102). Instead of dismissing the patient's request again, the doctor took 37 seconds of silence (Line 105) and rephrased his statement of rejection (Lines 106, 108), emphasising his understanding of the patient's difficulty (Lines 110, 112).

(25) Case 17, B: Silence and rejection

101	D	**It- it's >not a medicine that I can< give more of.** **One- The amount of the medicine is fixed. Um…** 増や- 増やすのはね (.) >できない薬なんですよ<. それは. 一つって- 量が決まってる薬なので. Um : .
102	P	**Look, it's not like I walk to the toilet, so** **it's right here, [so,** **So, I don't think you need to worry about that, but…** トイレほら : 行く訳じゃないから, ここにある [から, だからその点は安心だなと思うけど.
103	D	**[Yes. Yes. I see…** [う : : ん (.) う : : ん.そうですね : : .
104	P	**I'll leave the decision to you.** 先生のご判断に任せます.
105	D	**Hmm…** う : : ん. (37.0)
106	D	**I've taken another look at what medicines you're** **taking currently…** 今の, 飲んでる薬とかをもう一度点検して見てみましたけど : :
107	P	Yes. はい.
108	D	**Um… after considering the possibility of side effects,** **I wouldn't recommend using any additional medicine.** う : : ん. その副作用の可能性を考えると,そういう追加でお薬 を使うのは, 私はやめた方がいいと思い[ます.
109	P	**Right. I understand.** [わかりました.
110	D	**Right… well, I really understand how you feel.** **I think they turn the lights off early** (at the care home) **though (hh)** ((laugh)) う : : ん. まあ, お気持ちもよく分かりますし, 暗くなるのが早いなと思いますけど (hh),
111	P	**Yes.** はい.
112	D	**I bet it's not easy to sleep,** **£ even though they turn out the lights at 8 £.** **Um. But I think it's better to avoid it.**

£8時に暗くされてもね£.
なかなか寝れないなって，あろうかと思うんですが：，
う：：ん．おそらく，避けた方がいいと思います．
113 P はい．
I see.

I categorised this extract as empathic behaviour rather than an instance of *Works towards shared decision-making* (II.a), because they had already negotiated this request before this extract (see the full version of this transcript in Appendix 9.5) and the doctor needed to respond further to the patient's discontent with sleeping at 8pm at the nursing home. This task went beyond answering the patient's request for extra tablets; the 37 seconds worth of silence (Line 105) was used strategically to show the level of the doctor's understanding of the patient's circumstances. The doctor emphasised the pronoun *'I'* and the word *'avoid'* (Lines 108, 112), giving the recommendation on a personal level. In the post-consultation interview, the doctor briefly mentioned that he understood that those exchanges with the patient did not constitute a *'shared'* discussion:

> I deliberately use a paternalistic style occasionally. 'I won't prescribe it to you because it's not suitable for you', I do it like this. Like today's case, the patient who requested the sleeping tablets. I say, 'I understand your feelings, but I think this is best'. I don't reject them without reasons. [D3: Paragraph 13]
> あえてパターナリスティックにする時があります。「あなたには向かないから出しません」とか、そういう風にすることもあります。今日の睡眠薬のくだりとかね。あなたの気持ちもわかるんだけど、でも私はこうがいいと思うって。突っぱねたりはしませんけど。

There was a similar pattern of this for different doctors and patient participants. In Extract 26, the patient requested to stop taking the tablets that he had taking for the previous 10 years. The patient wanted to stop because he felt that they had not been effective. For the first half of the consultation, the patient's request to stop the tablets was persistent. The doctor convinced him first to reduce the amount of the tablets by slowly reducing the dose rather than stopping altogether (Lines 63, 65). In a similar way, as demonstrated by the doctor in Extract 25, the doctor in Extract 26 took 30 seconds of silence and eventually decided to stop the medication by accepting the patient's request (Line 68).

(26) Case 27, B: Silence and acceptance of the patient's request

56 P **Nothing has changed…**
I would like to stop taking medicines that don't work for me, one after another.
変わんね：：から，一応 (.) 変わんないのはどんどん切ってみようかなって．

57	D	**Well, it is fine to stop it, but,** あの (.) 薬をやめるのはいいんですけど,
58	P	**Yes.** はい.
59	D	**If you stop it abruptly,** 急にやめると,
60	P	Yes. うん.
61	D	**some people start feeling [pain.** 痛くなる人も[いるんですよね.
62	P	**[Ah, then,** [あ (.) じゃあ,
63	D	**Gradually, let's make it weaker.** 徐々に (.) 弱くしていきましょう.
64	P	**I see. Is 75 in the middle of…** はい. 75っていったら (.) 中,
65	D	**75 isn't strong, either. Let's make it <one level weaker.** 75も弱い方ですけども (.) < もう一段階 > 弱くしましょう. (30.0)
66	D	**I think 75 is weak enough for you, so…** 75で十分弱くなってるので,
67	P	**Yes.** はい.
68	D	**let's stop it this time, and,** 今回 (.) 中止にして,
69	P	**Yes.** はい.
70	D	**let's see how it goes.** 見てみましょう.
71	P	**Yes.** はい.

After the alternative suggestion *'let's make it weaker'* was made, both the patient and doctor remained silent. During the silence, the doctor was looking at the patient's history and confirmed that the condition of his liver was stable. It appears that the doctor made an attempt to understand the patient's request in further depth, before making the decision. Although the patient's description of his problem, such as why he wanted to stop the tablet, was brief (Line 56), the doctor attempted to respond to his desire, which was demonstrated with the silence. Extract 11 in Chapter 4 has also shown that silence may be used by doctors to show their empathy for the patients' situations.

Extract 27 is the last example of empathic silence, which emerged for each utterance throughout the consultation (Lines 35, 37, 39, 41). The doctor recognised that the patient often stated sadness and frustration about his debilitating long-term condition. The patient's tone of voice was one of frustration and irritation. The doctor spoke in a calmer tone and used silence evenly while phrasing his views. This appears to be a very careful attempt of displaying empathy.

(27) Case 26, B: Empathic silence between lines

34 P **I get irritated about myself, because I cannot move…**
自分が自分で (.) イ- イライラしてくるの. 動けないから : :
35 D **Ah,**
ああ,
(4.0)
36 P **Only my hands move, like this.**
手だけこうやって動くから.
37 D **Yes, yes…**
うんうん : :
(8.0)
38 P **When I lie down, my back hurts.**
寝てると腰が痛くなったりね.
39 D **Ah, I see.**
あ : : そうですね : :
(3.0)
40 P **All around my back is painful, and**
I feel like punching someone to get them to do something about it.
あちこちこう (.) 背中の方が痛いんで,なんとかしてくれって殴りたくなる.
41 D: **I understand.** ((sigh))
そうですよね : :
(5.0)

Although the patient seemed to be struggling to describe his feelings, the doctor waited until he spoke and engaged in less talking from her side. In the one-to-one interview with physician participant D4, she talked about the slow realisation that her communications with patients were ineffective because she was trying to persuade her patients through the use of medical knowledge rather than by listening to and understanding the patient.

> I used to rely too heavily on the verbal side a long time ago. Even though I studied hard to improve my verbal communication skills, I wasn't able to do it well, even using straight repetition. No matter how many times I used those techniques, they didn't work. I started thinking that it makes no sense to repeat while I'm still thinking that I want to persuade my patient somehow. [D4: Paragraph 7]
> 昔は、言葉に頼りすぎていたんだと思います。言葉をテクニック的にいろんなことを勉強しても結局うまくできなくて、おうむ返しにしましょうとか。いくらおうむ返ししても、結局どこかで説得してやろうみたいな意識の中でのおうむ返しは、しても意味ないのかなと思うようになりました。

D4 had decided to study philosophy at a graduate school while working as a family physician (a few years before this interview), and since then, she has specialised in the study of death, thanatology, as a subfield of philosophy. She stated that her interest in grief care has grown as she practices and that choosing the field of philosophy had come to her mind after going through many difficulties in interacting with patients:

> I found that it was important to think about what the patient is thinking in the background. I stopped thinking about little tricks for how to talk, and it turned out alright, as I felt able to do those little tricks at the end. Now I can express from my heart, 'I don't think so, but I see that you do think like that.' I have a feeling of respect for others who are different from me, like 'I cannot completely understand it, but it's been hard for you, right?' [D4: Paragraph 9]
> 背景にどう思っているかというのが大事だと思うようになって、その小手先のことを考えなくなったら結果的に小手先の事もできるようになったという感じです。「私はそうは思わないけどあなたはそう思うんだね」というのが自然に言えるようになった。自分と違うものに対する敬意のようなものができたんじゃないかなと。「私には完全には理解できないけどあなたも大変なんですね」という。

5.2 Potentially Non-PCC Elements

The following Extract 28 is an example of BEING JUDGEMENTAL (I.c.4). The patient fell at home five years ago, and recently broke her thigh bones and underwent an operation. At the beginning of the consultation, she told the doctor that recently she had been suffering from constipation and that this pain might have been caused by lack of exercise. Thus, she had worked in the garden. The doctor listened to her story for three minutes and exhibited impatience, providing advice not to do gardening anymore. The doctor's recommendation to the patient not to do gardening anymore (Lines 62, 64) may be interpreted as interfering judgement.

(28) Case 8, A: Interfering judgement

62	D	**<u>But</u> I think you've done well enough.** **When you work that hard on gardening=** <u>でもね</u>：：十分やられてるほうだと思いますよ.その (.) 庭の手入れなんて, そんな頑張ってやったらね=
63	P	**Umm…**
64	D	**=Your son would be worried about you, and,** **you may fall and break your bones again or become unwell or something like that, so,** **I don't think you need to work that hard.** =また息子さんも心配しているようにね,また転んで骨折したりとかね, 体の調子が悪くなったりとかね,するから, そんな無理にね, やらなくてもいいと思います. うん.
65	P	**I don't overdo it…**

		まあ無理はしないけどね：：
66	D	**It's not good when your stomach gets cold, either.** **You don't need to move your body that hard,** **but you can have hot meals,** **massage the area around your stomach,** **or take a bath that's not too hot...** 冷えとかもよくないですよね. お腹がやっぱり冷えてるとね, 体そんなに頑張って動かさなくてもね, あったかいものを摂るとかね, お腹マッサージするとか, 熱くないお風呂に浸かるとかね：：
67	P	**My stomach was always cold, before I became sick.** お腹は年中冷えてましたね, 病気になる前も.

The doctor attempted to persuade the patient not to work hard on gardening, which sounds restrictive. The patient seemed to hold back her thoughts and insisted that she could manage gardening (Line 65), which appears to be an attempt to preserve her face and the tone of voice sounded as if she interpreted the doctor's recommendation as interfering. However, the doctor tried to convince the patient, referred to the possible negative consequences of gardening, and provided the advice without connecting to the patient's feelings or emotion or acknowledging her stomach pain from constipation (Line 66).

Although it was uncertain whether or not the doctor was aware of this, she did not choose an indirect option but selected one without redressive linguistic action. This situation corresponds with the suggestion by Robins and Wolf (1988) that doctors could consider whether their words may damage the patient's face and could redress this by applying linguistic politeness strategies. This again confirms the benefit of integrating face concepts and PCC notions to produce a methodological tool fit for the analysis of medical consultations.

5.3 Empathy as the Core of Clinical Communication

As mentioned in Chapter 1, there is a strong correlation between how empathic communication skills are taught and the clinical examination OSCE in medical education. All the physician participants talked about how limited the time and scope of communication skills education was in medical school. Four out of the six physician participants explained that they only had opportunities a couple of occasions to learn how to interview patients in their fourth or fifth year of medical school and that the relevant educational materials were limited in the relevant assessment scope of OSCE. Two physician participants, who graduated before the implementation of OSCE, stated that they had not received any training related to the topic of communication skills or empathy. They expressed the opinion that teaching empathic communication with patients remains a great challenge in all medical schools in Japan. Physician participant D7, who was a recent graduate, recollected that medical student tended to feel confused with some of the phrases illustrated in the OSCE role-play materials:

> Basically, the so-called 'OSCE generation' uses this one phrase 'That must have been hard'. I do not use this phrase often. It feels sympathetic. But [in medical school,] everyone in my class was confused [when doing role-plays], because we all had to say that line and felt it may be rude instead. It does not sound caring. Empathy is more like identifying 'You think that …', right? Given that, what made us confused at that time was the sense that that ['That must have been hard'] was not the phrase to use. [D7: Paragraph 7]
> 基本的に、いわゆるOSCE世代は「それは大変ですね」ですから。僕はあまり使わない表現です。感覚としてはシンパシーです。それなのにその台詞を皆言うので、皆で混乱していたのです。むしろ失礼じゃないかと。他人事な感じがする。思ってないでしょって。エンパシーは「あなたはそう思っているんですね」になるんですよね。だとすると、学生の時に皆で違和感を感じていたのは、表現が違うってことですね。

This statement describes how educational materials apply sympathetic phrases in the broadest sense. Although such discussions on the interchangeably used expressions of sympathy and empathy are more common in Western literatures (e.g. Jeffrey, 2016; Soto-Rubio & Sinclair, 2018), D7 appears to suggest that sympathetic language in Japanese tends to sound rude, as they would connote a superficial understanding of the subject. In the Japanese educational textbook by Saito (2000), the author stresses that doctors should avoid expressing sympathy, because this may expose their patients to emotional stress (Saito, 2000: 52). The distinction between sympathy and empathy is rarely explained in those Japanese textbooks, although this could be associated with translation issues as well. Physician participant D2 also mentioned a cultural assumption that people tend to consider communication styles as 'ritual forms', which is based on his experience of assessing his students:

> Only the surface level of the concept 'empathic communication' is becoming prevalent. It's tested in the OSCE, so all students are thinking from the very beginning about where to put empathic statements in an interview, because they will lose marks if they don't appear empathetic. But there is no evidence. There is no evidence [in Japan] on whether the patients truly feel persuaded or satisfied with empathic remarks. In Japan, communication is a 'ritual form' like the tea ceremony, flower arranging, judo, karate, and so on. When it comes to talking about its hidden aspects, it becomes more religious. [D2: Paragraph 5]
> 共感的コミュニケーションと言われるものが一人歩きをしていって、学生達はOSCEの試験で出るので共感的態度を言葉を示さないと点が下がるんです。学生は皆、どこで共感的発言を入れようか最初から考えているん

> です。でもエビデンスがないんですよ。本当に共感的な発言をすると患者さんが納得するのか満足するのかどうかエビデンスがないんです。日本は、コミュニケーションは「道」ですから。茶道、花道、柔道、空手とか、型ですから。見えないところの説明になると宗教的になるんです。

The word 'ritual form' is used here to refer to the general cultural philosophy shaping Japanese communication style, which is supposed to encompass showing respect, empathy and compassion through the speaker's behavioural forms. Health settings include numerous traditional interactional behaviours performed in everyday life, greetings, bowing and placing both hands pressed together in front of the chest. These formulations have a social significance that is independent from what is said linguistically in most situations, not specifically health situations. D2 is also a practitioner as well as an educator and has authored textbooks on communication skills for young doctors. However, he mentions that there was a gap as he perceived it, between his understanding of communication and the demand from young doctors for 'quick fixes', e.g. universal tips on how to communicate. The greater demand to solve communication issues was exacerbated by the structural and contextual heavy workloads of doctors:

> It is difficult to know what to say to a patient who is in a really difficult situation, without learning through experience. [...] There is no answer. Well, there is an answer. You will ask why he or she thinks so and show empathy with the feelings. But this is only superficial. There is a huge difference between those who can find the right words to say and those who cannot as medical professionals, as people who provide care. [...] To some extent, it is partly based on skill and partly not. I stopped writing about teaching communication skills for this reason, because there were so many requests for 'tips' on how to communicate well. [D2: Paragraphs 10, 11]
> 本当に辛い状況にいる患者さんに対して何を言うかは、場数を踏まないとどう声を掛けるかって難しい。 [...] まあ答えなんかないですよ。一応ありますよ、なんでそう思ったのかを聞いて気持ちに対して共感してとか。でもそんなのは通り一遍のことで。そこでちゃんとした言葉がかけられる人とかけられない人で、医者として、ケアをする者としてだいぶ違いがあるじゃないですか。 [...] ある程度、スキルとスキルでない部分があるので。途中でコミュニケーションのことを書くのをやめたというのはそれに近くて、依頼がすごく多くて、こうするととてもうまいコミュニケーションができるみたいなのを皆求めていたんです。

He valued the logical connection between actual experiences in practice and the development of skills in that they can take into account cultural and social norms. On the other hand, some participants felt that it was extremely important to convey and teach young doctors theories of 'how to' communicate with empathy. D1 is also an educator while also practising as a family physician. He acknowledges the positive impact of the

Western-originated concepts and hopes to utilise the knowledge in his teaching in medical school:

> Since I have to teach medical students, I need to be a role model to some extent, so things like my professionalism have gone up. Also, the perspective of doing everything you can for the patient in front of you when practicing. After becoming an educator, I had to think about how best to convey that to a diverse group of students. If there is a student who can't do it well, what can I do to get them to learn it? In education, that sort of perspective comes in. There are several communication models and I have found that it's important to teach them in a way that's easy to understand. [...] I would like to use works of arts when teaching empathy, otherwise students will find it uninteresting or too rigid. It is better to cultivate the students' sensitivities through artworks and listening to real patients' stories. [D1: Paragraphs 15, 17]
> 学生に教えなきゃいけないので、自分が模範にある程度ならないといけないなっていう、プロフェッショナリズム的なものが少しだけ高まりました。あと現場にいるときは目の前の患者さんにベストを尽くすっていう視点ですよね。教育者になったあとは、それをどういう風に色んな人に伝えて学んでもらうかっていう視点があって、うまくできない人がいたとしたら、そういう人に学んでもらうとしたらどうしたらいいか。教育だとそういう視点が入ってきて、コミュニケーションのモデルというのがいくつかあって、そういうのをわかりやすく伝えていくっていうのも大事なんだなっていうことがわかりました。 [...] 共感を教える時にアートを使ったりしていかないと学生もつまらないし窮屈だと思うんです。アートに触れたり患者さんの話を聞く中で感性を耕していく方がいいと思うんですね。

Throughout the interviews, the physician participants demonstrated a strong interest in being educators alongside delivering practice, and in the extent to which educational and political concepts are being incorporated into teaching. Five physicians in this study have pursued their careers along those paths as a result of miscommunication in their own practice and the wish to reduce its occurrence in their consultations.

5.4 Conclusions

The doctors' approaches to the patients' emotions and feelings shown above appeared to be supportive and therapeutic behaviours that addressed the patient's positive face for the majority part. The communicative acts are grouped and summarised in Table 5.1. Some of the examples were, in fact, combinations of positive and negative face address. In other words, the professionals overtly displayed their willingness to help the patients and showed sensitivity towards the patient's feelings while at the same time giving the patients space to think. These subtleties are difficult to analyse as for example, the participants' non-verbal features could influence the whole discourse, yet these cannot be identified as

Table 5.1 Summary of the communicative acts in *Empathy and Acceptance*

Category of Face-PCC	Features
I.c. Displays empathy and acceptance	• EXPRESSIONS OF POSITIVE REGARD were the most frequent acts in the category of empathy. The professionals expressed empathy more explicitly in Consultations A, and willingness to help the patients (with pain or sad feelings) was overtly displayed. These included: ▪ Combination with giving some space ▪ Reassurance by including family ▪ Praising for doing well ▪ Positive regard and withdrawing judgement • UNDERSTANDING AND APPRECIATION OF THE PATIENT'S FEELINGS was used through a neutral stance (neither agree nor disagree with the patients' views) and included: ▪ Combining understanding and positive imagination ▪ Tuning the tone of voice to the patient's depression ▪ Picking up the patient's fear • Doctors may use SILENCE AS EMPATHIC ANTICIPATION to show their understanding for the patients, and these included: ▪ Silence and rejection of the patient's request ▪ Silence and acceptance of the patient's request ▪ Empathic silence between lines • A small laugh or smile heard in the tone of voice could soften the formality of the medical consultation • [Potentially non-PCC] BEING JUDGEMENTAL included: ▪ Interfering judgement

audio-recorded data. However, some aspects of non-verbal elements, such as longer silences, the doctor's light laughter or smile and tone of voice, were observed and duly coded. The data showed that these non-verbal acts can mitigate the formality, giving the statements made more personal significance.

6 Work Towards Shared Decision-making

The phase of shared decision-making concerns the degree to which the physician helps the patient to be involved in the discussion for possible treatment and to find a mutual understanding of the problems, medication and the patient's life context. This is achieved by statements that use concise, easily understood language, avoiding jargon; assessing the patient's starting point and values; using explicit signposting; information in manageable chunks, checking for understanding (e.g. *'Does that make sense so far?'*); sharing own thinking as appropriate; relating explanations to the patient's perspectives; and seeking collaboration (e.g. *'We will work together and try to sort time problem out'*). Stewart *et al.* (2014: 108) define reaching a mutual agreement as encompassing three key tasks: (1) defining the problem, (2) establishing the goals and priorities of treatment and (3) identifying the roles to be assumed by both the patient and clinician. By addressing the dimensions in the patient-centred communication (PCC) analysis, it can be possible to identify culture-specific aspects of involvement or independence that can be used to reach a shared understanding, agreement and decision-making in the medical consultations.

In most consultations with the presence of family members, the doctors spent more time explaining and planning treatment with the family members than with the patients themselves. The physician participant D7 explained that patients and family members participated in the consultation and that their stories were useful in gaining a clearer understanding of the patient's situation. He commented that, regardless of whether the setting was hospital or home, he always paid attention to the family perspective:

> In an outpatient booth [in hospital], if a patient comes with family members, what the family says is very important. In terms of focusing on the family's story, my communication style is not that different. When visiting a patient's home, the place, as well as the people there, offers advantages. But, in terms of non-verbal communication, there are differences between hospitals and homes, so I utilise any information I can. [D7: Paragraph 6]
> 外来のブースに座っていて、家族が一緒に来る場合は家族の話が結構重要です。コミュニケーションスタイルはそれほど違わないです、家族へのフォーカスという意味では。家に行けば、人だけではなく、場の利点もあり

ます。非言語的な意味でのコミュニケーションは病院と家では違うので利用できるものはします。

Visiting a patient's home has advantages that helps doctors to gain a deeper understanding of the patient's lifeworld, background and family circumstances, reaching a better shared discussion. Using non-verbal information to make better interpretation of their words being said during a consultation is a universal approach among medical teams whether at home or in hospital settings. The greatest difference between institutional and home settings might be the behaviours that are appropriate to the specific context (cultural performance): for example, at home, they would often take social roles as the hosts and guests.

6.1 Evidence of Work Towards Shared Decision-making (II.a.)

SHARING UNDERSTANDING (II.a.1) was most commonly performed in *Work towards shared decision-making* and was evenly seen in both Consultations A and B. SHARING THINKING (II.a.2), on the other hand, was more frequent in Consultations B (patients attending with their families and/or friend or neighbour) than in Consultations A (patients attending on their own). These results indicate that the doctors demonstrated explanations more overtly when the family was present. OFFERING SUGGESTIONS (II.a.3) was observed in three cases, respectively, in both Consultations A and B. It was especially noticeable that the professionals often avoided assertive attitudes towards the patient and family and softened their directives or possible dominance in the processes of decision-making. The opposite category, NO SHARED DISCUSSION (II.a.4), which was potentially non-PCC, was infrequent: two cases were identified in Consultations A and one in B. This aspect will be further discussed in Section 6.2.

6.1.1 SHARING UNDERSTANDING (II.a.1)

Extract 29 is an example of a situation in which the patient rejected the doctor's suggestion. The patient suffered from lung disease and chronic constipation, and the previous week he had received treatment for his bowels in hospital. At the beginning of the consultation, the doctor told him that she had examined the X-ray of his bowels. She had already suggested starting a new medication previously, but the patient respectfully conveyed to her that he was unwilling to try it (Lines 77, 79).

(29) Case 7, A: Not dismiss the patient's desire

76 D **I think >the movement of your bowel has been bad generally.< Umm...**
>全体的に腸の動きが悪いん<だと思いますね :: . うん :: .
(3.0)

77	P	**I see. Well, for the moment, I would like to continue like now, and see how it goes, rather than starting the new [medication.** だから, あの : : . ちょっと(.)今の形で,ちょっと : 様子を見たいなと(.)思ってですね : : 新しい薬じゃ[なくて.
78	D	**[Not yet. You would like to see how things go, still.** [はい. まだね(.)様子を見たい.
79	P	**Yes. That's what I think, but,** はい. 自分の考えはそうなんですけど,
80	D	**Yes.** はい.
81	P	**what do you think, doctor?** 先生はどうですか↑
82	D	**I was thinking that we would start trying the new medication, [though...** 私は (.) 新しいお薬を試してみようかな : : と思ってたんです[けど : :
83	P	**[Yes, but, for the moment...** [うん. もうちょっと : :
84	D	**Right, right.** うん (.) うん.
85	P	**That one I am using now...** 今のあれを : .
86	D	**Okay. Well, then, let's consult the care manager to see.** うん, うん (.) ちょっとじゃあ,ケアマネさんと相談してやってみましょうかね.

The patient's tone of voice remained calm and determined, and it seemed that he did not intend to start the new medication. After expressing his view, he said, '*What do you think, doctor?*', with an emphasis on 'doctor'. The plan for the medication had already been arranged between the patient and doctor, the local hospital and his care manager. Although the doctor did not dismiss the patient's desire to continue the current medication (Lines 78, 82), she concluded the discussion by using the inclusive form '*let's consult the care manager to see*' (Line 86). The care manager has overall responsibility for planning care for older adults in the local government; thus, they can intervene in the patient's care. The aspect is related to social practice – insurance-based care in Japan, which combines healthcare and long-term nursing care system.

Extract 30 refers to a combination of positive and negative face address used by the doctor to reach a mutual understanding. The patient had previously been hospitalised for a stroke and after discharge had undergone the aftereffects of the operation. Although the patient was trying to walk carefully so as not to fall, the doctor was able to elicit the information that the patient had stumbled occasionally (Lines 101, 103). The doctor's expressions softening the caution were specific: '*I hope that you would not fall if possible…'* (Lines 102, 104) just as a statement of hopefulness so that this advice did not sound too forceful and satisfied the patient's wish to act as independently as possible. The professional thus avoided asserting herself over the patient.

(30) Case 13, A: Softening the face threat in directives

97	P	**Well… after all, regarding a fall…** あの：：やっぱりね (.) 転ぶのはね：
98	D	**Have you often fallen?** 転んじゃってます↑：
99	P	**I try not to fall on my buttocks like before…** 前みたいに, お尻を打たないように：.
100	D	**£ You fall skilfully £.** ((laugh)) ((Use of humour)) £上手に転んでるん hh ですね£.
101	P	**It's painful when I fall on my buttocks, so I try to do it as little as possible.** ((laugh)) お尻うつと痛いので, なるべく打たないように hh はい hh
102	D	**I hope that you would not fall if possible…** なるべく転ばないのが (.) いいと思うんですけどね：：
103	P	**After all, my feet do not touch the ground properly,** やっぱり足の裏が (.) ちゃんと (.) 着地しないので,
104	D	**I hope that you make sure you're standing properly on the ground with each step…** 一歩一歩ね, ちゃんと着地を確認していただくといいんですけどね：： (2.0)
105	N	**You said that you tend to move in a hurry.** 慌てちゃう時が多いって言ってましたよね.
106	P	**Yes, I do.** そうですね.

During my fieldwork, all the physician participants stated that one of their greatest concerns was the patient falling, which could lead to the patient breaking their legs, having to stay in bed for a long period and losing physical strength. Thus, they repeated the caution in a softened manner. It can be difficult, however, for the professionals to advise the older patient to be careful in their daily activities after discharge from hospital, because many of them still wish to do their own things independently and doctors do not want to undermine their confidence that they can do so. Sometimes giving advice might sound forceful.

The focus of the patients is not necessarily the same as that of the doctor. This was more obvious when the respective participants used very different words. Extract 31 illustrates these contrasting thoughts with regard to what was the problem for the patient actually was. The patient's daughter and neighbour attended the consultation. Previously the patient had fallen several times, broken her hipbone and taken medicine for osteoporosis. The patient explained to the doctor that her foot had swollen and hurt. The doctor's focus was the result of her previous blood tests and whether they showed any internal problems. The patient, by contrast, talked at a great length (this consultation lasted for 42.8 minutes) concerning whether the cold compress she used to cure the swelling was working.

(31) Case 16, B: Different views of the problem

64	D	**You had a blood test last time, right?** **In the results, albumin, a protein element that indicates nutritional status, was <a little low.> I want to compare the data from the previous blood test you had. Do you have them?** この間ちょうど採血しましたよね. それでは,アルブミンっていって,栄養状態をみる, タンパク質 : の成分なんですけど,それが少し (.) <低め> ではあるんですが, 前の血液データって : : ありましたっけ.ちょっと比べてみたくて.
65	PF	**They must be here, right?** ((PF asks to P)) ここにあるよね↑
66	P	**I am wondering if this compress wouldn't work…** この湿布薬っていうのは : : 効かないものなんですか↑
67	D	**It's easy to get swollen when it's (albumin is) decreasing…** それが : だんだん減ってきてると, むくみやすいっていうのが : : ,
68	P	**Ah, I see.** あそうですか. […]
88	D	**Ah, it's getting better.** ((D checks the previous blood test result.)) あ (.) 少し良くなってきてますね. […]
90	P	**Doctor. Is that compress better than this?** 先生, オー湿布の方がいいんですか↑ […]
95	PF	**My mother says…** 母親がいうには : : ,
96	D	**Yes.** うん.
97	PF	**She said that a cold compress helped her swollen foot go down when she put in on her instep.** **Does a cold one work better when you put it here on your foot?** むくみ 足の甲に貼るのは (.) 冷たい方が腫れがひいたって言うんですよね. 冷湿布のほうがいいんですか 足のここに : 貼るの. […]
114	D	**Yes, it does, if her foot was swollen badly…** **It depends on where it hurts.** **>It's often said< that a foot may have swelling** **if your heart or liver or kidneys are bad.**

But her kidneys are not that bad from the results of the blood test.
うん (.) すごい<u>腫れ</u>ちゃえばね：. どこが痛いかですよね.あとは, >良くいうのは,<
心臓と肝臓と腎臓が悪くなると,足がむくんでくるんですけど,
腎臓は悪くないんですよ, 採血の結果で見るとね.

115 P **Right.**
ええ.

For the patient and daughter, the focus was on the cold compress, showing concern about whether it would work against her pain (Lines 66, 90, 97). On the other hand, the doctor concentrated on the results of her blood test throughout the extract, confirming that there seemed to be no problem with the patient's internal organs. The utterances of the participants do not seem to respond very closely to each other; instead, it even appears that in some sense they are participating in separate conversations. Although the patient, daughter and neighbour eventually felt relief after the doctor's diagnosis, it took about 20 minutes of interaction (the first half of the consultation) to reach common ground, i.e. that there was nothing to worry about in the results and to establish whether the cold compress was effective. This example shows an interaction in which patient and the doctor perspectives are different, and how the doctor spent time educating the patient, thereby reducing her concerns.

6.1.2 SHARING THINKING (II.a.2)

In examples of SHARING THINKING (II.a.2), the doctor spent time exploring the patient's values and provided explicit recommendations. Extract 32 shows how the doctor attempted to respond to the patient's request to remove his gastrostomy (gastric) tube from the stomach, by attempting to elicit the patient's thoughts. The patient had been hospitalised due to a cerebral infarct. His cognitive status was currently stable; however, it was difficult for him to move his lips. The doctor slowed down the speed of talk to match the pace of the patient's talk. His wife and son did not attend the consultation, because the patient had shown displeasure at the fact that the professionals discussed his medication only with his family. The patient asked why he could not remove his gastric tube and expressed his wish to have it removed. The doctor asked why he was wanting this (Lines 54, 56) and suggested that he should keep it in for the time being in order to maintain his good physical condition for a long time (Line 58). Throughout the conversation, the doctor paused frequently.

(32) Case 14, A: Willingness to support the patient's autonomy

54 D **If it's okay for you, I would like to ask you about (2.0) why you want to remove the gastric tube.**

(2.0) Whether we remove it or not, the food you eat
by mouth will not change.
もし良かったら (.) 伺いたいんですけれども,
(2.0) 胃ろうは, 閉じても閉じなくても (.)
口から食べるもの, については, 変わりないんですけれども,
(2.0) どうして閉じたいとか (2.0) 理由はありますか↑

55 P (inaudible)

56 D **When I asked you last time,**
(2.0) you said that you wanted to try
any methods that give you a chance to stay well
and live longer.
Do you still feel this way?
以前, 伺った時に (2.0) 出来るだけ, 元気で長生きできような方法を,
なんでも試したいと, 仰ってましたけれど, 今もそのお気持ちと,
変わりないですか↑

57 P **I still do.**
変わりはありません.

58 D **This is my suggestion. (2.0)**
It will be easier for you to stay well and live longer if you keep the gastric tube, as it brings enough nutrition to the body. (3.0)
It would be better to keep it. This is my opinion.
これは, 私からの提案なんですけれども, (2.0)
胃ろうがあったほうが, 体に十分, 栄養がいって, 元気で長生きしやすいんですね.
(3.0) 胃ろうは,あった方がいいんじゃないかな, というのが, 私の意見です.

59 P (inaudible)
((P concerned that his family had decided his treatment without consulting him.))

60 D **Since I first met you, I have tried to explain to you**
as many times as possible in person, and
I have tried to choose the best option by consulting you,
(2.0) not by talking to your son.
I always want to know how you feel.
初めてお会いした時から, 私はなるべく, 色んな事を, (patient's name) に直接
説明しようと思ってますし, (patient's name) のお返事 (2.0) を聞いて,
一番いい方法を, 選んできたつもりなんですね.
息子さんと相談するとかじゃなくて,
ご本人の気持ちを 知りたいっていう風に思っています.

The audio-recorded patient's responses were drowned by the noise of an air cleaner beside his bed, but the doctor was able to listen to him and spoke distinctly and slowly. The doctor understood that the patient's concerns were not merely about his gastric tube but also about decisions made by his family without consulting him. The patient desired his autonomy with regard to his treatment. The doctor showed willingness to be supportive for the patient and shared opinions with him, respecting his wish to be independent (Line 60).

Some cultural differences could be argued in relation to a decision-making process. D2 expresses the view that cultural differences must be always included in the discussion, because this issue can be profoundly associated with cultural norms:

> Americans praise their children so much, you know, saying 'My kid is the best'. Those who look critically at us Japanese people say that Japanese parents do not praise their children or nurture their self-esteem. Certainly, there are cultural differences, and let's say, cultural relativism. We don't hug each other every time we meet in Japan, do we? The number of international workers has increased in Tokyo in the past 10 years, and the way of thinking has diversified. It's been changing, noticeably when giving bad news. Until about my fifth year as a fully-fledged doctor after finishing as a resident, delivering bad news to cancer patients was never an option in Japan. Now, we do almost 100% of the time. However, there are some traditions left, such as informing family members of it without the patient's agreement. [D2: Paragraphs 6, 7]
> めちゃくちゃ褒めるじゃないですかアメリカ人は、オーバーにうちの子供はナンバーワンだって。批判的に見る人は、日本人の親は子供を褒めないし自尊心を育てないと言う。文化相対性主義もありますけどやはり違いはあると思います。日本では会うたびにハグする文化はないです。ここ10年東京では外国人が増えて、考え方も多様になっていますし、とくに変わったのは告知のところです。僕が研修医から医師になって5年目くらいまではがんの人に告知するなんてなかったです。今は、ほぼ100%します。ただ本人の同意を得ないで家族に話すとか、そういうところは今も残っています。

Some approaches that were unheard of 20 years ago have become common in Japan, one of which is telling the truth to cancer patients, for example. When introducing the concept of informed consent, Japanese medical educators have added more advanced skills such as breaking bad news, giving information to the patient and addressing the patient's emotions. This has accelerated the adoption of patient-centred concepts, as prior to this change, patients were not well informed about their illness or even not involved in a decision-making process.

The next extract shows a discussion between the patient's family and the doctor. In Extract 33, during the discussion, the patient was present but not involved. The patient lived alone, but her daughter usually attended the consultation and discussed the patient's medication with the professionals, which was a common situation in most of the data. The patient had suffered from pneumonia, and after being discharged from hospital, she was struggling to walk. The doctor reported the results of her blood test to her daughter to discuss the prescription. The report included some bad news, and the doctor's expressions were mostly indirect, and the daughter's responses were very short.

(33) Case 22, B: Reporting results to the family

21	D	**Well, her kidney function is not very good, but…** すこ ： ： しだけ (.) 腎臓の働きが, よろしくないんですけど : :
22	PF	**Ah, right.** あ (.) はい.
23	D	**Let's say… as long as she takes care of it** **more carefully than a young person would,** **her kidney would be fine for the next 10 to 15 years.** ま : : 若い人と比べて (.) 少し (.) 大事に使えば, 10年 15年もちますから.
24	PF	**Right. I [understand.** あ (.) はい. 分かり[ました.
25	D	**[Let's think about the future after that at the right time.** [その先はそれで考えましょう.
26	PF	**Right. I understand…** はい (.) 分かりました : :
27	D	**Also, the indication for heart failure is marked 'high'** **but if the indication is under 500** **it is not particularly [problematic…]** あと, 心不全の指標も, 高いっていうマーク付いてるんですけど, 500以内であれば (.) とくに, [問題に]なるような心不全ではないので : ,
28	PF	**[Ah], I see.** [あ.] そうですか.
29	D	**I don't think it's problematic.** 問題がないと (.) 思います.
30	PF	**I see.** はい.

As mentioned above, such an interaction is common between the family and the doctor, in which the results of a blood test are reported, and the doctor's assessment discussed. The doctor appeared to choose the modifier and vagueness (Lines 21, 23, 25) so as not to worry the family, which led to little response from the family (Lines 24, 26, 28). This part shows that the family – not the patient – was informed of the doctor's knowledge and encouragement.

Family participation was not always so passive; some cases included the more active involvement of family members. The last example of II.a.2 SHARING THINKING, Extract 34, shows how the family's opinions could influence the process towards shared decision-making. The doctor observed the progress of the patient's recovery who had been hospitalised due to a leg fracture. When the doctor asked the patient's preference regarding tablets (Line 102), the patient's husband (PF-H below) and daughter (PF-D) immediately cut in (Lines 103, 104), suggesting that she should reduce the amount of tablets.

(34) Case 28, B: Family involvement in decision-making

98	D	**Well, your condition seems good when you take the tablet.** まあ (.) 飲んでて調子がいいので,
99	P	**Yes.** はい.
100	D	**You can continue to take it, or…** このまま飲み続けるっていうのでもいいですし：,
101	P	**Ah, I see.** あ (.) そうですか.
102	D	**you can reduce or stop it. What would you like to do?** 減らしたり止めたりもできますよ. どうしたいです↑
103	PF-D	**We'll see her condition again [and…** もう一回様子 [見て：,
104	PF-H	**[Stop (taking the tablets) this time,** [一回とめて,
105	PF-D	**Do we [stop it?** 止め[ちゃう↑
106	PF-H	**[Let's see her condition.** [様子見て.
107	D	**Let's see how it goes…?** 様子見て. ((D asks P))
108	P	**Yes.** はい.
109	D	**Then, let's see and discuss again if we can stop or reduce… we'll consider it.** 様子見て, ちょっと相談して (.) また止めたり, 減らしたり：, 検討していきましょう. […]
113	PF-H	**We can ask to get the tablets again if something is wrong. You had better reduce it as much as possible.** ((PF-H talks to P)) なんかおかしかったら (.) また足して貰えばいい. なるべく減らした方がいいよ.
114	PF-D	**Do we reduce the tablets? And let's see for two weeks and we can ask to get prescription again if something is wrong.** ((PF-D talks to P)) 今回減らす 減らして, 2週間見て,次の時にまたおかしかったら, も一回出してもらえばいいんじゃない↑
115	PF-H	**Yes. That's better.** そうだね (.) その方がいいよ.
116	P	**The pain is severe when my stomach hurts…** 半端ないもんね. お腹痛くなるとね：
117	D	**Right… when it hurts.** うん：：なった時が,

The husband and daughter believed that the patient should reduce or stop the intake of her tablets and their intervention appeared almost forceful. During this discussion, the doctor handled the situation by talking to the patient directly to confirm if it was acceptable with her, *'Let's see how it goes...?'* (Lines 107, 109). It seemed obvious that the patient was concerned about the pain and still would take the tablets, as mentioned *'the pain is severe when my stomach hurts'* (Line 116), but she did not explicitly mention so. They concluded by agreeing to reduce the amount of the tablets rather than stopping altogether. While the male patient in Extract 32 had a stronger desire to participate in decision-making, the female patient attending with her family in Extract 34 did not necessarily expect to have the same level of involvement in decision-making.

6.1.3 OFFERING SUGGESTIONS (II.a.3)

The extracts in the previous category above have included examples of OFFERING SUGGESTIONS (II.a.3) as well. The patients and families rarely asked the professionals for clarification about the information provided, and their obedience, which would be assumed as culturally expected, could potentially prevent the professionals from obtaining an understanding of the patient's needs or concerns about plans and treatments. Although the professionals certainly applied their knowledge in those interactions, moving towards shared decision-making seems to be a skilful interactional task that requires communicative skills.

Extract 35 is an example of offering options that seems prescriptive, explicitly applying negative politeness strategy. The patient became unwell after taking antibiotics and stopped taking them after three days. The doctor switched her task from taking a history to educating the patient on antibiotics (Lines 166, 182, 188), which led to the patient admitting her mistake *'I was careless...'* (Line 189). They reached an agreement, after a three-minute-long process that included clarification, education and offering options.

(35) Case 4, A: Prescriptive advice

166	D	**Your previous doctor. Did he tell you that** **once you start taking it, you need to take it for** **seven consecutive days and finish it?** **Were you told that?** これ前の先生にはね (.) 先生には, 1回飲み始めたら, 7日間で飲みきるようにって言われませんでした↑言われてない↑
167	P	**He <u>might</u> have said that (hh).** ((laugh)) おっしゃった (hh) <u>かも</u>しれない.[...] [...]
179	P	**After I took the tablets for three days,** **my stomach felt heavy, and I didn't feel like eating anything,** **[I just slept.]** あの 3日間飲んでたら[ね, 胃が重苦しい感じがして,] なんかなんにも食べたくないし, [で寝てたんですね.]
180	D	**[Right, right.]**

[うんうん, うんうん.]
[…]
181 P **So, I thought it was no good to keep taking them.**
だからこれじゃあダメだろうと.
182 D **Yes, I see. There are some side effects.**
With medicine, if you stop taking it partway through,
well, have you heard of 'resistant bacteria'?
うんうん, そうですね. それなりに副作用もあるし, お薬をね,
こう中途半端に飲んでしまうと, 耐性菌って聞いたことあります↑
183 P **I haven't.**
知りません.
[…]
188 D **This means that if you plan to take it, you should**
take it properly for the whole week, and,
if you don't plan to take it fully, you should take
none at all. Meaning, either zero days or seven days
is the way to do it, so,
飲むんだったら一週間しっかり飲んだほうがいいし,
のまないんならもうのまないどっちかですね.
ゼロか7日間かっていう感じでね(.)やったほうがいいので,
189 P **I was careless.**
不注意でした.
190 D **No, no. It's no problem, no problem at all.**
I just think we should try it like that next time.
いえいえ(.)いいんですいいんです. そういう風に今度から,
しようかなって思うんですけど.
191 P **Yes.**
はい.
192 D **Then, shall we try just water next time?**
If you don't have a stomach-ache or any symptoms like that,
just drink water even if you have blood in your urine=
そしたら次回は, お水だけでやってみます↑特にお腹痛いとか
症状なければ,
血尿出てもお水だけ飲んで=
193 P **Yes.**
はい.
194 D **=without taking antibiotics, shall we try that?**
=抗生剤はのまないで, やってみます↑
195 P **I'll try that.**
やってみます.
196 D **Let's do it.**
やってみましょうか.

Negative politeness strategy is salient throughout this extract. Towards the end of the discussion, the inclusive forms such as *'we should…'*, *'shall we…'*, *'let's…'* were frequently used (Lines 190, 192, 194, 196). This hedging seems to be used to minimise the communicative pressure on the patient in pointing out the mistake of the use of antibiotics.

The previous extracts have also shown a similar tendency, where the professionals softened their assertiveness of suggestions.

6.2 Potentially Non-PCC Elements

Extracts 36 and 37 are examples that combine NO SHARED DISCUSSION (II.a.4) and DIRECTIVES (II.b.3). The doctor reported the result of the patient's blood test and calcium level to the patient's daughter. In the co-presence of the patient, the doctor delivered her knowledge on how to improve the situation and handed out a prescription, without including the patient.

(36) Case 22, B: Focusing on the doctor's knowledge (example of II.a.4 and II.b.3)

32	D	**The level of calcium is a little... low...** カルシウムが少 : : し低いかな : :
33	PF	**That's right. She takes the medicine for calcium once a month, which I get from the [clinic.** そうですね. カルシウムの薬は月に一回飲んでますね. クリニックで頂いてる[やつ.
34	D	**[I think it's one that reduces the level of calcium.** [逆に下がっちゃうやつだと思いますそれ.
35	PF	**Eh, really?** え (.) ほんとに↑
36	D	**Medicine for bones, right?** 骨の薬ですよね↑
37	PF	**>Yes, that's correct.<** >うんそうそう<.
38	D	**Because it takes calcium into the bones,** **the level of calcium in the blood is reduced.** あれは, 骨のほうに持っていっちゃうんで, 血液中のが減っちゃう.
39	PF	**Ah I see.** あそうなんだ.
40	D	**Yes, it's better for her to take a separate calcium supplement or some medicine that helps improve calcium absorption...** うんだから (.) 別にカルシウムを飲むとか, カルシウムの吸収をよくするお薬を飲んだほうがいいんですけれど : .
41	PF	**I see. Hmm...** そうですか. ふ : : : ん. [...]
47	D	**Well, vitamin D, to begin with,** **From food, um, use vitamin D...** **there is a medicine that helps absorb calcium from food better.** **She will take one tablet per day=** とりあえず, ビタミンD, 食べ物から : , えっと (.) ビタミンDを使って,

食べ物から, カルシウムの吸収を良くするお薬があるので,それ
一日一粒 : =

48 PF **Right.**
うん.

49 D **=I will prescribe it from here.**
=出しておきます (.) こちらから.
[...]

60 D **To begin with, I would like her to take the vitamin D medicine,**
just one per day.
まずはちょっと : ビタミンDのお薬を, 一日一粒だけ, 飲んでもらおうか.

61 PF **Right.**
はい.

The doctor provided the result and explanation simultaneously and quickly progressed to problem-solving (Lines 40, 47, 49, 60), in which there can appear no shared discussion. The issue is that there is little room for the daughter to think and her responses were very short, and the flow of decision-making and control appears to follow the doctor's directives. In this case, the participants would potentially miss an opportunity to work on shared discussion together.

Similarly, Extract 37 also shows a missed opportunity for shared discussion; this is, however, caused by the patient's initiative. The patient stopped taking a medicine in the mornings without telling the doctor. The doctor explained the disadvantages of stopping it, in a way that attempted not to be judgemental about the patient's decision.

(37) Case 11, A: Missed opportunity to a shared discussion (example of II.a.4; II.b.3)

1 P **This medicine- my stool was just awful every day,**
so I stopped taking it just in the mornings.
(2.0) Since then, it's been better.
この薬- 便の出方がね : : 毎日毎日ひどかったので, 朝だけちょっと,
やめたんですよ. (2.0) そうしたらよくなってきたので.

2 D **This medicine?**
この薬ですか↑

3 P **Yes, yes.**
ええ, ええ.

4 D **I see.**
わかりました.

5 P **I know it's not good to stop it entirely,**
so I only stopped that much. It gets better now.
全部やめるとよくないので, これだけやめたら,よくなってきましたので,

6 D **Ah, I see. Do you know >what this medicine is?<**
ああ (.) そうですか. これ実は, >なんのお薬かわかります↑<

7 P **Well, in short, the medicine is for urine…**
I thought that, so I thought it might also work for bowel movements as well.
なんか : : 要するにあれだろ, あの尿の, 関係. そうだと思ったので,
便にもいいのかなと私は思ったんだけどね.
[…]

13 D **I see. I cannot say there is no relationship between this medicine and stool. But I cannot say that they're absolutely related to each other.**
((potentially preventing the patient from articulating his view))
なるほど. 関係は絶対ないとは言えない. でもそんなに : :
目立って関係があるとも言えない.

14 P **Ah, I see.**
ああ, そうなんですか.

15 D **If there are any problems from stopping the medicine,**
it could become harder to urinate, and
at the worst, urine could accumulate without coming out…
これをもし減らして, 弊害があるとすれば,おしっこが出にくくなって,
一番ひどいと, 出たいのに出なくて溜まってきて : ,

16 P **Right, right.**
はいはい.

17 D **It's called "urinary obstruction".**
ということですね. 尿へいっていうんですけど.

18 P **I don't have that.**
そういうことはないんですよ.

19 D **Normally it might be okay to stop it.**
Shall we try, then?
((no shared discussion))
普段はそれでいいかもしれませんね : . それで試してみましょうか↑

20 P **Right. I thought it would be good to do so.**
そうですね. そうしてもらえたらいいかなと思ったんです.

This consultation displays the patient's initiative at the start (Line 1), and it can be seen that the patient expected the doctor to be receptive towards his decision. However, the doctor's strategy was to test the patient's knowledge about the medicine (Lines 6, 13), providing information and the risks of stopping the medicine (Lines 15, 17). Although the doctor eventually agreed, it seems that the patient did not intend to change his mind (Line 20) and exercised control over this conversation. Here, the doctor's behaviour is not necessarily perceived as directive or dominating, as the doctor stepped back into his knowledge to negotiate an appropriate pattern of decision-making. The comment *'Shall we try?'* indicates that the doctor does not wish to impose on the patient, but similarly to Extracts 36, the quick problem-solving could also prevent the patient from articulating their views.

6.3 Challenges of Shared Decision-making as a Young Doctor

Physician participant D1 shared his story that he was urged to acquire skills to talk to patients and families when working as a resident physician, especially after a patient complained about his tone when delivering explanations:

> I was in charge of a patient with cerebral infarction. In general, these patients all vary regarding how severe the damage is and how much after-effects remain. So, the patient and his family were very anxious. I was in the second year of my residency, and I had to explain to the patient's wife by myself. I thought I tried my best, but she got even more worried about the situation. It became an issue and I had to bring the head of the neurology department in to explain to the patient's wife and son again. Thinking about it now, it was because of the way [subtle difference] I had spoken. I should have spoken accurately but without causing anxiety in the listener. There are situations where a resident doctor should not be left to talk to a particular patient [or family] alone, which I know about now but didn't know at that time. [...] Looking back now, I think what you learn in the first few years is really integral, and whether you can learn basic communication skills in the first few years as a resident doctor will affect you much later. Unfortunately, I had no opportunity to take a formal class on the subject, and as a result, I ran into difficulties in real-life experience [due to insufficient knowledge of the communication skills]. [D1: Paragraphs 3, 4]
> 脳梗塞の患者さんがいて、どのくらいのダメージなのか、後遺症がどのくらい残るのかとかは千差万別なので、患者も家族もすごく不安なんです。僕が研修医2年目のとき、僕一人でその患者さんの奥さんに説明をしました。僕は一生懸命説明したつもりだったんですけど、奥さんがそれで一層不安に思ってしまって。息子さんと神経内科の部長を含めてまたもう一度説明しないといけない事態になったんですね。今考えると、微妙な話し方のせいなんです。正確なことを話しつつも、不安を持たせない話し方っていうのもある。この患者さんには、研修医一人にさせてはまずいとか、今だったらわかるんですけれど、当時は分からない。 [...] こうやって振り返ってみると最初の数年間での学びというのはすごく大きくて、研修医になって最初の数年間のうちにしっかりと基礎的なスキルを学べるかがあとまで響くと思います。僕は残念ながらコミュニケーションのフォーマルな授業は受けなかったけれども、それで実際に困ったという経験が沢山ありました。

He explained that a subtle difference in the way he had spoken resulted in anxiety for the patient's wife. He then reflected that the issue was the need to convey information as accurately as possible and to mitigate the patient's and family's worries. Doctors gain an awareness of how particular skills could work in real-life consultations during their residency programmes. All the physician participants said that they began to learn the communication skills required in practice on their own. A large part of their narratives focuses on the challenge they endured as young doctors, which led them to change the way they talked to patients and families.

These events included their own direct experiences or the accounts of other doctors in the same workplace or other settings, indicating that the notion could be influenced by the way in which it is used in their institutional discourse.

6.4 Conclusions

Overall, the skills for shared decision-making included a greater use of negative politeness strategies rather than positive politeness. Positive politeness involved addressing the patient's name, showing willingness to support, and sharing opinions, whereas negative politeness involved respecting the patient's wish to be independent, use of particular inclusive forms and expressions of hopefulness, softening the offers that were frequently observed. Some patients desired autonomy, and some did not necessarily wish to decide. The communicative acts are grouped and summarised in Table 6.1. As mentioned in Section 6.1.1, the Japanese context involves more intervention by multiple occupational roles based on the national insurance system. This inevitable element in the intervention can be extremely influential for a decision-making process for the patient's care.

Table 6.1 Summary of the communicative acts in *Works towards shared decision-making*

Category of Face-PCC	Outstanding features
II. a. Works towards shared decision-making	• The doctors' acts included greater exercise of negative politeness, and they demonstrated the process of shared decision-making more overtly when the family was present. SHARING UNDERSTANDING included: ▪ Not dismiss the patient's desire ▪ Softening the face threat in directives ▪ Different views of the problem • Some patients desired their autonomy with regard to medication, whereas others appeared to defer to their doctors' recommendations. The acts of SHARING THINKING included: ▪ Willingness to support the patient's autonomy ▪ Reporting results to the family ▪ Family involvement in decision-making • OFFERING SUGGESTIONS could also be seen as: ▪ Prescriptive advice • The family's opinions could negatively influence the process towards a shared decision-making • The inclusive forms *'Shall we...?'* are often used to soften a request and mitigate the doctors' DIRECTIVES. The potential non-PCC acts included: ▪ Focusing on the doctor's knowledge ▪ Missed opportunity to a shared discussion

7 Leave Space for the Patient and Respecting the Patient's Freedom

This chapter illustrates physicians' responses that leave space for patients and show respect for their freedom. These aspects are at 'the heart of respect behaviour' and particularly concerned with social conventional styles. They occur in situations in which a balancing of power is required, because it performs the function of minimising the imposition on the patient. One particular cultural aspect was related to *physical touch* and *proximity – closeness/distance*.

7.1 Evidence of Leaving Space for the Patient (II.b)

Since the professionals needed to cover information of the patient's problems, other issues the patient wishes to tell and benefits and risks of the medicine in a short amount of time, they hoped the patients would understand their explanations. CHECKING FOR UNDERSTANDING (II.b.2) was seen as a brief summary of the explanation on prescription, and the doctor asked if the patient had any questions. Few of them, in fact, took the time to check the patient's understanding or address misunderstandings. Six cases were identified in Consultations A (patients attending on their own) and five cases in Consultations B (patients attending with their families and/or friend or neighbour). Second, OPEN QUESTIONS THAT OCCUR THROUGHOUT THE SESSION (II.b.1) was infrequent, only two cases in Consultations A and one in Consultations B, although they were semi-open enquiries to keep the patient talking.

7.1.1 CHECKING FOR UNDERSTANDING (II.b.2)

The purpose of checking for the patient's understanding was to simply avoid a minor mistake of the prescription that had been agreed with the patient and/or family. The patient usually answered *'yes'*, and a further question hardly ever occurred.

In Extract 38, the patient's family always joined in the consultation, and most of the interaction occurred between her family and the doctor.

After discussing prescription with the patient's brother and his wife, the doctor summarised the session.

(38) Case 21, B: Confirming prescription

187	D	**Today, I'll <change> the prescription a little bit.** じゃあ今日はね, お薬をちょっと少し<変えますね.>
188	P	**Ah, I see.** ああそうですか.
189	D	**Because I don't want your foot to get infected with bacteria, I'll give you an antibiotic and a stronger medicine to relieve swelling.** バイ菌が足についていると嫌なので, 抗生物質と, ちょっとむくみをとる薬を強くします.
190	P	**Ah, I see. Thank you.** あそうですか(.)はい. よろしくお願いいたします.
191	D	**Do you have some of the ointment [left over?** ((D asks PF)) あと塗り薬は余りは[ありますか↑:.
192	PF	**[We use it. Well,** [塗り：薬は付けてます (.) あの,
193	D	**>Today I'll give you another ointment, which you can put on her toes. I'll also give you eye drops, just in case.<** ((D talks to PF)) >今日もう一個, 軟膏, これあの足の指のところに付けて, 目薬も念のために出しておきますので.<
194	P	(3.0) ((silence))
195	PF	**Because someone familiar visits us now like this, we feel very relaxed.** 今ね, こう：顔なじみの方が来てくれるので, すごくリラックスしています.
196	D	**£ Ah, I'm glad to hear that £.** £ ああよかった £.

The doctor could have made some attempts to check the patient's understanding; instead, the doctor confirmed the change of the prescription (Lines 187, 189, 193). These utterances appeared to function as a signposting and the closure of the consultation, for which the family member seemed to relax and thanked the doctor (Line 195).

Similarly, Extract 39 shows that the professionals commented on the patient's new bed when closing the session. In a relaxed mood, the doctor asked if there were any other problems at the end of the consultation.

(39) Case 20, B: Final checking

145	D	**Now you've got the new bed…** とりあえずベッド変わったことでもね：：
146	N	**I think your rehabilitation is going to be much easier.** ずいぶん楽になると思う (.) リハビリも,

147 D **I agree. I think the care will be easier to do, too.**
Do you have any other problems : : ? [Are you okay?
そうですね. ケアもしやすくなると思います.
あとなんか困ったこととか : : [大丈夫ですか↑
148 P **[No, no. I'm fine.**
[いや, ないです. 大丈夫です.

The final checking (Line 147) was also signposting of closing and space for the patient to clarify their own terms. Checking for understanding (II.b.2) is important for patients in terms of having more freedom to talk or ask questions. However, only a few patients made much use of this opportunity, and the interaction mostly ended with a one-way transmission from the professionals.

7.1.2 OPEN QUESTIONS THAT OCCUR THROUGHOUT THE SESSION (II.b.1)

Ensuring space for the patient could have been made by OPEN QUESTIONS THAT OCCUR THROUGHOUT THE SESSION (II.b.1), which was infrequent. Open questions can be used to give more space to the patient to talk at some length as shown in the following extracts. Extracts 40 and 41 illustrate open or semi-open questions used in the middle of the consultations.

(40) Case 9, A: Semi-open enquiry while checking the condition

13 D **Keep your hands relaxed.**
手はね, 楽にしててください.
(42.0)
14 N **36.3 degree.**
6度3分です.
15 D **The temperature is fine.** ((writing a record))
Your legs may be swollen because your kidneys are like that [though.
お熱も大丈夫ですね.腎臓があれだから, 足むくんじゃうことあります[けど.
16 P **[Well…**
[あの : :
17 D **(How is it) recently?**
最近は↑
18 P **The swelling has mostly gone away.**
むくみはね, だいぶとれた.
19 D **Ah… they look fine. There is no particular change, right?**
I'm sorry, let me check the other leg.
((checking her foot))
あ : : 大丈夫そうですね. 別段とくにお変わりなく.
反対側の足もごめんなさいね.
(3.0)
20 P **I wasn't able to wear shoes when I was young.**
若い時なんか, 靴履けなかった.

The patient seemed to want to talk and stated '*Well…*' (Line 16), and the doctor immediately made facilitative responses, '*recently?*' (Line 17) and '*There is no particular change, right?*' (Line 19). This appeared to show that the doctor noticed her wish to talk and gave her some space to do so, and she began to tell her story (Line 20).

In Extract 41, the doctor asks about the patient's lifeworld at the beginning and end of the consultation. While the nurse was checking the patient's vital signs, the doctor read his record and showed his interest as to how the patient's wife had been – she was living in a nursing home. The doctor asked a general enquiry to the patient's son later on. The topic of the family member seemed to play an important role in that the professionals could notice any changes to the patient's circumstances. This could also facilitate the smooth transition to further focused enquiries.

(41) Case 17, B: Asking about the patient's lifeworld

12	D	**By the way, I haven't seen your <wife> recently.** **Is she still the same as always?** そういえば私最近, <奥様> お会いしてませんけど, 奥様の方も (.) 特別お変わりは,
13	P	**Yes, I don't think anything's changed.** ないと思います.
14	D	**I see. That's good.** そうですか (.) 何よりでした. (6.0)
15	N	**98, 83.** 98, 83.
16	D	**98, 83.** ((writing it down)) **Have you been able to <eat> well?** 98, 83. <お食事は>しっかり食べれますか↑
17	P	**Well, now, I've been asking for my rice to be cut down** **to about 70% of what it was.** そう：ね：今ご飯をね, 七分目くらいにしてもらってるんですよ. […]
153	D	**Do you have any concerns? Is everything okay?** ((asks to P's son)) 息子さん何か, 気になってらっしゃることとか. 大丈夫ですか.
154	PF-S	**It's fine.** 大丈夫ですね. (2.0)
155	D	**Sounds like everything's okay.** ((encouragement)) 特になさそうですね.

The doctor initiated by expressing implicit interest, stating '*By the way, I haven't seen your wife recently*' (Line 12) rather than asking directly about how she had been. Indirectness was used as a conventional linguistic formality and hedging when asking about the family members.

In addition, the enquiry to the patient's son, *'Do you have any concerns? Is everything okay?'* (Line 153) did not include any specification, leaving the question open and waited for a couple of seconds.

7.2 Evidence of Respects the Patient's Freedom (II.c)

7.2.1 Linguistic deference (II.c.1)

LINGUISTIC DEFERENCE was often seen as extra indirectness to mitigate the force of task priorities for the patient's negative 'face-wants' (a specific desire to be unimpeded in one's actions), which was identified in four cases in Consultations A and one in Consultations B. This also included giving apologies for touching the patient's body. In Extract 42, the thermometer sounded a signal, and the doctor made an indirect comment, *'the thermometer seems to have beeped'*, to notify the patient of taking out the thermometer. The patient did not hear what the doctor said and the doctor made the same comment again. The doctor was standing in front of the patient and was trying not to impose the action. In the end, the resident physician stated the request more directly (Line 4) and helped the patient to take out the thermometer.

(42) Case 2, A: Giving a hint

1	D	**The thermometer seems to have beeped.** もう鳴ったみたいです (.) 体温計.
2	P	**I see.** そうですか.
3	D	**The thermometer seems to have beeped.** 体温計鳴ったみたいです.
4	RD	**Shall we take the thermometer from under your left side?** 体温計取っちゃいましょうか (.) 左の脇の.
5	P	((takes the thermometer)) (6.0)
6	RD	**Excuse me. 36.4 degrees.** 失礼しますね. 36度4分.

It appeared that the doctor did not wish to perform any verbal or nonverbal FTA here (Lines 1, 3). The resident immediately intervened, as the patient might have been waiting for the professionals to help him or had not heard. This intervention by the resident did not just assist the patient but also could be an act to save the doctor's face, as it might seem that the patient had ignored the doctor.

Another example, Extract 43 shows that the doctor often used the word *'seem'* with a terminal patient receiving palliative care to inform her of how refreshed she looked on that day (Lines 172, 174). The doctor also used a linguistic form of respect for the word *'appear'* (Line 176). In fact, the use of the word *'you seem…'* was extremely common in the doctor's statement in all the consultations.

(43) Case 10, A: Deference through the use of 'seem'

172	D	**You seem to have recovered (from depression). Yes, yes.** 少し持ち直しましたね. うんうん.
173	P	**I have.** 持ち直して.
174	D	**£ It seems so from your facial expressions £.** £ 表情からも, そのような : £
175	P	**Are they different?** 違う↑
176	D	**£ Yes. It appears so £.** £うん. お見受けします£.
177	P	**hhh** ((laugh)) **Sorry… I'm being selfish : :** hhh ね. わがまま言って : .
178	D	**No, no. Please let me know how you feel again.** いえいえ. またお話聞かせてくださいね.

Lastly, the professionals used particularly indirect forms to request permission or acknowledging discomfort when touching the patient's body. In Extract 44, the doctor explained what was to be checked and asked permission to do it with a linguistic form of respect for the word *'if I checked'* (Line 42) along with the modifier *'a bit'*. The nurse also expressed sympathy about removing the patient's clothing, mentioning that she was aware of how cold it was that morning (Line 43). No response was given by the patient during the check.

(44) Case 20, B: Asking permission for touching the body

42	D	**Last time, there was a part on your skin around here** **that had turned a bit red.** **Would it be okay if I checked <a bit>** [whether it's returned?] この前このへんが, 少し赤くなっている所があったので, またそれが[ぶりかえしたりしていないかどうか,]〈ちょっと〉 見せていただいてもいいでしょうか.
43	N	**[I'm sorry.] I'm sorry : : that you must be cold.** ((moving the patient's clothes)) (2.0) **It was cold this morning.** [ごめんなさい]. ごめんね : : さむいところを. (2.0)今朝 (.) 寒かった.

In general, professionals' apologies about removing the patient's clothing or touching the patient's body were extremely frequent in all the consultations; this was often followed by the shorter statements such as *'Excuse me' or 'Let me check…'*. In addition, only the doctors' linguistic form often shifted to a form of respect in asking permission as shown above (Line 43).

7.3 Potentially Non-PCC Elements

The final Extract 45 shows an example of TOUCHING WITHOUT ASKING (II.c.2). This is the only example of the patient's reaction towards touching without asking permission (Line 61). For other potential cases, the patient did not react, and it is unclear if it negatively affected their communicative tasks or not. The patient suffering from pain in his back and legs shouted when the doctor touched his leg. The doctor used semi-open questioning regarding his leg, followed by five-second silence (Line 60). It was clear that the patient's reaction was a refusal to be touched.

(45) Case 26, B: Touching without asking

60	D	**How's swelling on your leg? Hasn't it changed much?** (5.0) 足のむくみとかはどうですか (.) あんま変わんない↑
61	P	**>It's painful when it's touched!<** > 痛いんだよ触られるの. <
62	D	**I am sorry. Which one has stronger pain?** すみません. どっちが痛い↑(2.0) (2.0)
63	P	**<About the same.>** <同じくらい.>
64	D	**About the same. Is it painful here as well?** 同じくらい. こういうところも痛いです↑
65	P	**It's painful.** 痛いね.

Touching the patient's body in a medical context can be perceived as discomforting or disturbing culturally. Asking permission before touching was a very common demonstration during the physical examination in all the consultations, in which the patient was informed of the forthcoming touching by either the doctor or nurse as shown in Extract 44.

In Japanese culture, hugging is not practised and social touching in general is mostly avoided, and even more so in healthcare settings. Some patients would expect the professionals to be aware of this sensitivity and the fact that being touched is not simply painful but also may cause emotional discomfort (Crezee & Asano, 2016). Therefore, there could be some contradictions between the social custom and PCC acts, although the act of touching itself is not taboo. It is simply required for professionals to ask permission to touch in order to materialise PCC in Japanese settings.

7.4 Conclusions

Throughout the consultations, the professionals' efforts to ensure space and freedom for the patients were captured by a variety of conventional indirect acts. It would not be easy to address all the problems they might have during the consultation, but it could make difference to add one more question for a check in order to check whether anything could be prioritised. The professionals' extra linguistic polite forms were occasionally observed. The physician communicative acts are grouped and summarised in Table 7.1.

Table 7.1 Summary of the communicative acts in *Leaving space for the patient* and *Respects the patient's freedom*

Category of Face-PCC	Outstanding features
II.b. Leaves space for the patient	• Final checking and affirmative statements functioned as CHECKING FOR UNDERSTANDING. These included: ▪ Confirming prescription ▪ Final checking • OPEN QUESTIONS THAT OCCUR THROUGHOUT THE SESSION included: ▪ Semi-open enquiry while checking the condition ▪ Asking about the patient's lifeworld • [Potentially non-PCC] DIRECTIVES was seen in the sequence patterns of a shared decision-making (in 6.2)
II.c. Respects the patient's freedom	• LINGUISTIC DEFERENCE was often seen as extra indirectness to mitigate the force of task priorities. These included: ▪ Giving a hint ▪ Deference through the use of 'seem' ▪ Asking permission for touching the body • One example of [Potentially non-PCC] TOUCHING WITHOUT ASKING was seen.

8 Transferring into Future Training

This final chapter revisits the aims of the linguistic analysis and discusses the future potential transfer to professional training, as well as the use of the Western-originated model of patient/person-centredness in different cultures.

8.1 The Relevance of the Home and Family Context

The patient-centred communication (PCC) communicative acts *Displays empathy and acceptance* and *Works towards shared decision-making* were most commonly seen in the data. The salient feature of empathic skills is that they are grounded in the doctors' capacity for carefully listening to the patient, picking up cues and responding appropriately. Showing understanding for the patient's views and feelings by turning the patient's pessimism into a positive view tended to be followed by describing favourable outcomes. It was also commonly seen that the professionals showed their interest in the patient's family at the beginning of the consultations.

In Consultations A (patients attending on their own), the professionals tended to initiate closed questioning that immediately followed up a problem from the previous consultation. In Consultations B (patients attending with their families and/or friend or neighbour), on the other hand, the doctor tended to spend a few minutes to establish common ground with the family by applying semi-open questioning, which allowed the professionals to wait for the family to take the initiative in terms of raising the specific concern of the patient. This difference explains the infrequency of the category, GRADUALLY MOVES FROM OPEN TO CLOSED QUESTIONS (I.a.2) in Consultations A. A similar contrast can be seen in the sharing thinking category. The doctor provided explanations more overtly to family members or third parties than to the patients attending on their own. This finding suggests that the task priorities and sociability were flexible, indicating more participation when the family was present. This has important implications for practice. Another feature often observed was that the professionals tended to gain more information about the patient (problems and contextual background) from the family than from the patient themselves, and therefore the family's opinions may significantly influence the course of the consultation, more importantly, the process of shared decision-making between the participants, and less participation of the patient.

Yamaguchi *et al.* (2016) discuss the perspectives of family caregivers with reference to the points raised above. The authors' qualitative data indicated that family members often looked after the patient at home, not simply because they were family, but because they voluntarily wished to do so and were willing to participate in caring. At the same time, socio-cultural expectations meant that they were pressured or even forced to perform this social role, particularly felt by females. The authors noted that family decision-making reflected the strong bonds inherent in family relationships, specifically with regard to the doctor's prognosis and end-of-life care. These aspects have also been clearly shown in the data in this study. The findings in Consultations B show families adopting these social roles, which are also associated with the doctor engaging in more spontaneous social talk.

The family's sense of responsibility on behalf of the patient may reflect a general cultural tendency. It is a way of protecting the patient from potential emotional suffering and pain caused by the sharing of bad news. Family decision-making can reduce the challenges of family care at home. However, the patient's wish for family members' involvement in decision-making varied considerably. Ten out of 14 patients in Consultations A lived with family but voluntarily chose to attend the consultation on their own, in a separate room from the family. There is always the possibility that family involvement could result in the patient's unwillingness to talk about their lifestyle, ideas and thoughts about treatment plans, which could also impact the realisation of doctors' PCC acts.

8.1.1 The impact of family involvement on consultations

Involvement of family and further interventions by third parties is increasingly incorporated to support the older adults receiving care services. The physical presence of family members and other professionals for the patient's care in one single consultation is therefore not uncommon, and there is the expectation that their opinions will be equally appreciated. All the physicians interviewed indicated that they opt for a family or group-oriented style and that their patients are generally on the whole happy for family members to be with them when the physician discusses their diagnosis and treatment, although some will want privacy and autonomy in decision-making. The overall findings from the Face-PCC features show that the presence of family members has more complex impact on the consultation, especially on the doctor's open and semi-open questioning, empathy and the process of decision-making.

Although the physician participants described dealing with family members as most challenging particularly in their early careers, family members' stories were always appreciated by the professionals. For example, Participant D7 explained that he tended to see the family's opinions as very important and that he adapted his consultation style according to the setting; specifically, he spoke of 'tuning in' to family opinions if they were expressed. Being in patients' homes was advantageous in terms of gaining a deeper understanding of the patient's lifeworld and circumstances. Regardless of whether the notion of patient-centredness is spoken explicitly, this doctor's positive interest in the patient is clearly patient-centred.

Particular cultural assumptions also need to be taken into account when discussing the development of consultation skills. D2's perception is that culturally Japanese patients do not express much emotion in interactions, compared to Westerners. In the traditionally collectivistic culture, medical professionals are expected to allow patients 'space' in their interactional behaviours. This results in the use of expressions aimed at addressing negative face and is particularly noticeable in the cases when doctors deal with patients' emotions.

Five of the doctors interviewed reported that they used to feel constrained by the 'diagnostic model' they practiced during their residency in terms of how they could respond to their patients' emotional distress. Since becoming family physicians, their perspectives had gradually shifted to the communication styles that is possible within the role of family physicians. They felt able to address the patients' anxieties by showing empathy; indeed, the possibility of a different kind of doctor–patient relationship was partly what drew these participants towards the career of a family physician.

8.2 Empathy and Related Strategies

Another outstanding feature was empathy – the common use of EXPRESSIONS OF POSITIVE REGARD (I.c.2), which was also detected in Backhaus' (2017) linguistic investigation of communication in an elderly care home. His cross-cultural comparison, using Brown and Levinson's (1987) politeness strategies, concluded that giving praise, including joking, was used frequently. In addition, he found significant similarities in the use of positive politeness strategies with the use observed in a previous study that analysed communication in a German nursing home, a UK geriatric hospital ward and a caring institution in South Africa (Lanceley, 1985). In this study, the doctor's EXPRESSIONS OF POSITIVE REGARD were the most frequent PCC acts in both Consultations A and B.

Backhaus' (2009) early study included not only verbal expressions but also non-verbal signs of praise, such as handshake for greetings by caregivers as a means of expressing positive politeness. In this study, on the other hand, I observed that handshakes were extremely rare and that the medical teams appeared to have taken a stance on the patient's sensitivity that touching the patient's body could cause discomfort. In terms of physical touching in a social and cultural context, a handshake is not unusual in a business context in Japan but is not customarily performed in other social situations. Indeed, this can be considered as an exaggerated expression of positive politeness, especially outside of the business context in some cultures. Supporting this stance, the doctors in this study, almost always used statements and asked permission such as *'I am sorry'*, *'Excuse me'* or *'Let me see...'* before touching.

Turning to the instances of cases for displaying empathy, when coding consultation strategies, empathy and REPETITION, PARAPHRASING AND INTERPRETATION (I.b.1) were frequently seen as combined. One utterance was normally coded for one skill (such as 'paraphrase of the patient's last phrase'), considering the stage of the consultation (such as 'a stage where the doctor initiates to retrieve information from the patient to take history'). However, a unit of discourse can encompass multiple functions – the doctor's listening techniques can also sometimes function as 'appreciation' and 'encouragement' at the same time, potentially requiring double coding for skills categories. From this point of view, the doctor's empathy and acceptance were often combined within their repetitions and paraphrasing, when listening to the patient; it was rather rare for listening to be demonstrated without empathy. This approach to the patients' emotions and feelings corresponds to PCC as set out and outlined the ideal steps illustrated in the Western model. Demonstrating listening skills – REPETITION, PARAPHRASING AND INTERPRETATION – appeared in harmony with the frequent facilitative comments made by the doctors. Thus, consistency between the literature review and actual practice of PCC acts can be found in the instances of empathy that occurred with the listening techniques.

8.3 Politeness Strategies

In existing literature, an orientation towards positive politeness strategies in the doctor's responses to the patient's utterance was noticed. The Face-PCC findings, in fact, confirm that doctors made wide use of mitigation strategies – negative politeness strategies, allowing patients and their families some space to express their opinions and make their own decisions.

Initially, the process of shared decision-making was expected to include sequence patterns of the doctors attending to the patients' positive face, including acknowledging their feelings and thoughts, encouraging the patients to engage with the process. It seemed relatively straightforward to identify the point where the doctor began the process of a shared decision-making, due to the doctor's clear signposting. Coding allowed me to confirm that the PCC-relevant skills were seen and that the patient and family responded with extra politeness to the professionals. The Face-PCC analysis highlighted that multiple positive and negative politeness strategies were adopted, increasing the complexity of the analysis. It was more significant that the professionals often avoided assertive attitudes and attempted to soften directives and provided 'room' to choose; these strategies ended up including a greater exercise of negative politeness rather than positive politeness in the phase of shared decision-making: respecting the patient's wish to be independent, the statements of hopefulness and softening offers. Both the structure and language of the consultations appeared greatly formal and fixed, thus adhering to the cultural expectations outlined in the literature. Overall, the professionals were observed adopting an attitude of respect towards older patients rather than familiarity. Due to these features and their frequency, *Works towards shared decision-making* was classified as a subcategory of *Attends to Patient's Negative Face*. These findings indicate that doctors' actual use of PCC may vary considerably according to a cultural context. Generalisations, therefore, need to be carefully considered with regard to the interactional conventions of particular cultures and settings.

8.4 The Calgary-Cambridge Guide and Cultural Diversity

The Calgary-Cambridge Guide (Silverman *et al.*, 2013) has been widely utilised in a variety of educational and professional contexts and not only within the teaching of communication skills (Ammentorp *et al.*, 2014; Greenhill *et al.*, 2011; Hammond & McLean, 2009; Nikendei *et al.*, 2011). In this book, the adoption of the model in non-Western countries, specifically in Japan, was considered with regard to interactions between older patients and physicians. It was noticed that the general structure of the actual consultations was organised by the doctor's clear signposting and followed the ideal structure as defined by the Calgary-Cambridge model, indicating that at a structural level, the consultations adhered to the model. The uniqueness of the context – in-home medical consultations – lies in the tasks that doctors are required to fulfil in order to meet the patient's needs in the setting. The in-home medical consultation requires healthcare professionals to engage in communication in the most personal environment where patients (and their lifestyle) are seen for longer than in an institutional setting.

Silverman *et al.* (2013) explore the application of particular communication skills in socially different communicative contexts. Communicating with older patients is listed as a special consideration in the Calgary-Cambridge Guide and is introduced by referring to Wolff and Roter's (2012) findings that being accompanied by family members was associated with indications of less patient-centred care. Specific challenges were associated with meeting older adults' needs, and both patients and physicians contributed more to the task-oriented and biomedical discussion. It seems particularly important for the doctors to encourage the patient's participation in their enquiries, building relationship by demonstrating sensitivity, empathy and support, and information-giving by clear signposting. In this study, I did not gain an impression that the doctors engaged in less question-asking, even though they used many closed questions with the patients and prioritising biomedical explanations; but overall, they appeared to be engaging in more non-medical conversations when the patient's family was present. When talking to the patients with a hearing impairment, the professionals strived to speak more slowly, distinctly, repeating particular words that the patient had uttered so as to give the patient the chance to focus their attention on the topic. The doctor's negative politeness strategies have also been interpreted as related to the cultural expectation of showing respect to the patient so as to reduce emotional discomfort. Thus, these more personalised settings with older patients seemed to enable professionals to find redressive actions and allowed more freedom in the patient–doctor relationship.

Communicative issues are listed in the Calgary-Cambridge Guide as common barriers in cross-cultural settings and social diversity (Silverman *et al.*, 2013: 235). While I do not address these wider aspects of cross-cultural communication, I highlight the aspects that appeared to be specifically relevant to the setting of in-home physician consultations in this study:

Use and interpretation of non-verbal communication

- Physical touch
- Proximity – closeness/distance

Cultural belief and healthcare

- Gender and age expectations about roles and relationships
- Role of doctor and social interactions related to power and ways of showing respect

Sensitive issues

- Uneasiness regarding some physical examinations
- Sharing bad news

Medical practice issues/barriers

- Extent of doctor/patient partnership, extent of family involvement, personal and family responsibility for healthcare and treatment

The seven aspects listed above were salient in this study. All the professionals paid special attention to physical touch and proximity, and the data show that letting the patient know when they were about to be touched was common to almost all the consultations, whether by the doctor or the nurse. Only one example was identified when permission was not sought, and the patient reacted accordingly, as presented in Section 7.3. The doctors were aware of the asymmetrical power relationship and the need to redress that asymmetry to some extent by showing respect through appropriate forms of address and seeking permission when conducting physical examinations. It indicates how important it is for professionals to act in conformity with cultural expectations and understand the patient's point of view when striving to engage the patients and achieve an interactionally optimal consultation. These elements can be taken into consideration when developing communication skills training in health and social care.

8.5 Physician Perspectives

During the one-to-one interviews, I asked six physician participants whether their communication style towards patients had changed since graduating from medical school, and if so, how and why they thought it had changed. The participants expressed emphatically how limited the time for and scope of communication skills education were in medical education. Two experienced physicians mentioned that teaching communication skills remains a challenge in all medical schools. All the participants spoke of learning through their everyday practice. They explained that as a group of professionals, biomedical views used to be predominant. However, in the past decades, through their practical experiences, the removal of patients' anxieties has become more of a priority. There was a shift from the biomedical model to a more 'psychosocial model'. The physician participants discussed a range of issues related to family involvement, interpersonal and interprofessional interactions, and cultural and social aspects. They all spoke of their awareness that the patient's family, and the opinions of family members are often considered more important than they used to be in the past.

Some physicians value having opportunities in their everyday practice to develop a variety of consultation skills, while others expressed the opinion that it is extremely important to teach young doctors 'how to' acquire specific skills in medical school, before they begin full time practice. The former position appears to assume that young professionals will learn through experience and threw drawing on conventional and social behavioural norms. The latter position, which highlights the importance of teaching consultation skills, acknowledges the positive impact of the Western-originated models and the value of applying the knowledge to teaching.

8.5.1 Professional mindset

All the interviewed doctors raised the topic of how they related communication challenges to the professional mindset. The most experienced physician among the participants, D2, perceives that his basic style of communication with patients has remained consistent, although he has developed advanced skills, including telling the truth to the patient.

Given that the experience of the physician participants ranged from 10 to 25 years of practice, I was also able to consider whether there were any observable differences in communication styles that might be linked to the doctor's age and experience. I gained the impression that their expressions during the consultation, as well as the perspectives and reflections they shared during the interview, were the belief that doctors must bring the patient a sense of comfort or relief and that the physician must gain the patient's trust. Considerations of cultural traditions have not been neglected in the international context of academic publications. My observation coincides with Matusitz and Spear's (2015) findings from comparative studies in the US and Japan, in which they emphasised that Japanese patients felt that their role was to obey and that the doctor should take on the leading role in the consultations. I would add that other cultural elements could include normative gestures in decision-making such as respecting the patient's ideas and actions in order to avoid conflict.

One factor that reduces the potential for PCC, according to the physician participants, was limited time – the ratio of talk in time constraint. They felt that this approach further increases the burden on the doctor, on top of the already heavy workload in clinical practice. All the physician participants agreed that time constraints in hospital settings were the greatest obstacle to adopting a PCC approach, even when they wished to do so. It was commonly mentioned that listening to patients requires considerable time and that in those settings it was hard to find enough time. All the interview data from the doctors included statements that many doctors in hospitals who were too busy looking at electronic medical records and did not appear to be paying much attention to the patients. D8, however, found that reducing the ratio of talking became a key point in improving his performance and making patients feel more listened to:

> In hospital, I tended to follow treatment models, which occupied my mind and the contents of what I said. Patients expected it too to some extent. With home visits, my communication style leans more towards looking at the patient's lifestyle. [...] My specialism was diabetes the whole time I was in the hospital, and now I do home visits looking at general internal medicine. The patient's background is important, so I listened to it to a degree, but I had to see so many outpatients and only had three minutes for each patient. It was not enough time to touch the patient or listen to their heart, and I just looked at the data and wrote the record. Now, I visit four or five patients in the mornings, but when I had to see 30 patients in the hospital in the mornings, I couldn't listen to them, even though I wanted to. [...] At first, I did not like the situation, but through handling the workload from necessity, I learned how I could make the patients feel satisfied even in a short time. Until then, I often focused on giving the information I wanted to tell, but I decided to reduce the ratio of talking as much as possible [and listened more]. This turned out well. Even though I really wanted to say something, I didn't say it if the

patient was not ready to listen to me, and I spent more time listening instead. Otherwise, the patient would have no chance to speak during the three minutes. [D8: Paragraphs 1, 10, 11]
病院にいる時は医療モデルになりがちなんです。自分のマインドも喋る内容も。患者さんもそれを期待している部分もあります。在宅医療はより生活モデルに近いコミュニケーションの仕方になるかなと思います。 [...] 病院にいるときはずっと糖尿病を専門にやってきて、今も内科全般として在宅を見ているという形ですね。実際に社会背景も大切なので聞くことは聞くんですが、とにかく患者さんが多いので、外来は3分間くらいです。体にも触れないです。胸の音を聞く余裕もないですし、データだけ見て、カルテを書いて。在宅だったら午前中は4人か5人を診ますが、糖尿病の外来で30人診るとなると聞きたくでも聞けないですからね。 [...] 最初はそういう短いのが苦手で嫌だったんですけど、必要に迫られてやってるうちに、短い時間でもどうやって満足してもらえるのか意識するようになりました。それまではこっちが話したいことを伝えるっていうことが多かったんですけれど、それを極力減らしたらうまくいくようになりました。本当は言いたくても、相手が聞く準備ができていなかったら、言わないでむしろ聞く時間を増やす。そうじゃないと相手も3分間何も話せないで終わってしまうので。

Participant D8 favoured short consultations, stating that since becoming the director of a clinic, he spent less time in consultations and that patient satisfaction was nonetheless always high. In this study, the average duration of the consultations was found to differ according to experience and gender. The consultations by experienced doctors were shorter, compared with ones by less experienced doctors. The average duration of the consultations involving the three experienced doctors (with over 20 years' experience) was 16.8 minutes, while it was 18.4 minutes for the five younger physicians (less than 14 years' experience). Regarding gender differences, the duration of the consultations with the five male physicians was 14.4 minutes on average and 22.6 minutes for the three female doctors. Thus, male physicians with more experience spent the least amount of time in the consultation. The difference in duration associated with gender was more significant than the difference associated with years of practice. It was noticed that female doctors spent more time having conversations with the patient and family than male doctors, and the average difference was seven minutes. D8 explained that it was crucial to him to reduce the ratio of him talking so that the patient felt listened to. It can be said that the issue is not the length of the consultation but whether the patient actually feels listened to. This could not be checked as part of this study but could be considered in further research.

8.6 Western Communication Models: Theory and Practice

Western theories about the patient–doctor relationship, especially the concepts and theories of patient-centredness, have played a significant role in introducing the principles of clinical communication skills worldwide.

Educational materials are designed to teach students the basics of interviewing skills; however, it was found that there was little indication that the theories were being incorporated into the students' learning in the classroom. In Japan, the contents of the actual training are left to each medical school, and the scope for teaching the Western models is currently limited to the requirements of the Objective Structured Clinical Examination (OSCE) assessments. Physician participants D1 and D2 emphasised that it has remained a challenge for educators to identify how to teach Western models of clinical communication in the medical education context. Some schools with wider programmes apply more role-play scenarios and supply students with references to the literature. The point could be whether consultation training has been nationally unified, and if not, this may widen the differences in the quality of individual doctors' practice. This could be less the case in the UK and US settings, as Western educators adopt a more standardised communication skills training approach in order to minimise significance of differences in practice of care (Brown, 2008; Kurtz *et al.*, 2003).

The physician participants had encountered situations of miscommunication with patients during their residency programme, which was attributed to the lack of training on how to communicate with patients and handle specific challenges. They began learning about the skills that are required in real-life consultations after becoming a doctor, through their own experience. In social care settings, different organisations can be involved in the medical care of a patient, and therefore, a number of professionals may be trying to provide appropriate care for a patient – this requires negotiation and cooperation, and all these professionals bring different perspectives according to their roles. This is one of the reasons why the medical teams openly share the consultation with other participants (family members or professionals), based on the social assumption that the patient would wish to do so. Conventional behaviours performed in everyday life are often considered as more important than what is stated verbally. As a result, junior doctors are more likely to employ socially accepted behaviours (redress politeness strategies) rather than cultivating specific consultation skills that are necessary for effective and patient-centred consultations. It seems, therefore, that it would be beneficial for young professionals to be supplied with more educational resources covering more substantial features of PCC, because accessing useful materials was identified as an issue.

8.7 Linguistic Politeness as Educational and Analytical Tools

By integrating medical and linguistic categories in the Face-PCC analytical framework, I was additionally able to integrate the observational data with the empirical findings, thus providing a social context for the linguistic analysis. This approach enabled me to explore the relationship between patient-centred features and cultural factors from a wider perspective.

In an early study that used the concepts of face and linguistic politeness in patient–doctor encounters, Robins and Wolf (1988) argued that the value of the approach was that medical students could achieve optimal patient-centred interaction by becoming familiar with linguistic politeness and other theories borrowed from the field of linguistics. The authors found that first-year medical students with no classroom training in medical interviewing skills tended to use culturally sanctioned politeness forms – negative politeness strategies – to repair communication, with linguistic behaviours borrowed from their everyday interactions, some of which were culturally appropriate, but not necessarily therapeutic (Robins & Wolf, 1988). They asserted that the politeness strategies described by Brown and Levinson illuminated culturally appropriate ways of communicating in medical consultations, especially with regard to doctors' noticeable difficulties in discussing the physical problems deriving from illness and disease. Negative politeness is most closely associated with notions of polite behaviours. In this study, the face-oriented approach casts light on a similar 'avoidance' tendency exhibited by the doctors and equally vague responses from patients, as emerged in the early studies (Robins & Wolf, 1988; Spencer-Oatey, 2007; Yin *et al.*, 2012). As those early studies showed, medical consultations are complex interactions in which participants assume different social roles and devote themselves to face maintenance. By merging the notions of positive and negative face with PCC elements in this study, I was able to observe the degree to which the discourse was therapeutic in practice. The category of non-PCC represents the potential for expressions that overtly threaten the patient's face. The interpretation is, however, highly context dependent. For example, the doctor's recommendation to the patient not to do gardening anymore may be interpreted as interfering judgement, and therefore, as potentially non-PCC (presented in 5.2). The doctor states: '*Your son would be worried about you. You may fall and break your bones again or become unwell, or something like that. I don't think you need to work that hard*'. The patient replies: '*I don't overdo it…*'. The patient's initial response appears to be an attempt to preserve her face and the tone of voice sounded as if she interpreted the doctor's recommendation as interfering. The doctor's advice was a request not to do gardening, and it was directly uttered.

Research by Yin *et al.* (2012) identified a doctor-centred pattern in a Chinese context, which invited further interest as to whether this might be observed in other Asian contexts. Their comparison of frequencies of politeness strategies showed that most of the politeness strategies used by paediatricians were bald-on-record, direct and non-redressed in consultations. In contrast, parents used more positive politeness and off-record strategies. This is consistent with descriptions by Brown and Levinson

(1987) and Morand (1996, 2000, 2003) that high-powered speakers in a situation are likely to use more bald-on-record strategies, while low-power speakers would use more off-record strategies. Yin *et al.*'s (2012) study included observations of triadic interactions between doctor, parents and children, which could potentially share features with other Asian cultures. In the Face-PCC findings of this study, negative politeness strategies were found to be frequently used by Japanese doctors when they were considering the patient's wishes, as a way of displaying empathy, or as a means to protect their patients' negative face.

Spencer-Oatey (2007) explained that theories of identity suggest that face has a number of characteristics that need to be held in dialectic balance. In this study, face was socially constituted in the particular interactions by their professional motivation. The patients had their 'patient face' which might be different from the face that they adopt in other communicative contexts. In the medical context, their responses may be more passive than in other contexts, as they rarely raised objections with the doctor. The patients appeared to be satisfied with the doctor's signs of interest. While the findings in this study have confirmed some of the findings from previous studies, as discussed above, the data have also shed light on the multiple aspects of the face concept: face is an extremely complex and multi-faceted phenomenon. As pointed out by Scollon *et al.* ([1995] 2011), face is understood as both 'involvement' and 'independence', and these two aspects do indeed appear simultaneously, which was the main methodological challenge in terms of analysing discreet communicative acts.

8.8 Summary

This study was designed to combine the concepts of PCC and Face with mixed methods to shed new light on the contextual aspects that shape the interactions. Conducting the observations and analysing the audio recordings turned out to be a suitable and workable method to obtain findings that could be cross-referred with findings from the fieldwork and linguistic analysis. Locher (2015) acknowledges that the scope of pragmatic analysis has been increasingly widened by approaches to politeness that include methodologies used in other non-linguistic disciplines. This means that the field of linguistics is now confronted with a wider range of data types and may be enriched through the insights gained from different methodologies, such as mixed methods of ethnography and interviews and/or focus groups. This study represents an example of this approach and has illustrated the benefit of integrating PCC communicative acts within face-relevant categories for the analysis of medical consultations. In particular, the inclusion of the face categories has cast a light on the feature of conflict-avoidance.

The physician participants were not necessarily confident that Western PCC concepts are clearly defined or workable and believe that any improvements in medical consultation practice need to take into account the needs of patients. Sociocultural expectations often mean that family members feel pressured or even forced to take on the social role and act on behalf of the patient, which clearly reduces the patient's participation. Interactional cultural preferences also shape the use of Face-PCC relevant expression, which was evidenced by the findings that the professionals often avoided assertive attitudes and attempted to soften their DIRECTIVES. The more personalised setting with older adults further could require the professionals to adopt redressive expressions and more formulations that address patients' negative face.

Finally, the application of the integrated framework of Face-PCC has highlighted the importance of considering cultural variations in the analysis and interpretation of face wants, and the extent to which strategies of positive and negative face are context-dependant. The multiple qualitative methods of integrating the findings of literature review with empirical investigation in this study constitute an important theoretical contribution, while they also highlight relevant methodological challenges in developing a context-specific analytical framework and interpretations of findings. The analysis has given a voice to the participants, highlighting the professionals' linguistic acts with regard to the patient-centred approach, and this ensures that the data are grounded in their experiences and practices within authentic consultation settings.

8.9 Contributions of This Study

One of the main contributions of this study is that it developed a methodological tool for analysing medical consultations in a culturally specific context. Although many empirical studies of communication in a health context have been increasingly conducted through qualitative approaches, the reliability of coding the data in a cultural context often remains opaque, due to interpretation issues. It was important to ensure that the analytical categories of this study were based on the literature review of both Western and Easy Asian publications and that the categories captured the verbal dimensions of the consultations, because the data only involved audio-recorded samples and my field notes. Transcription and translation were involved before initiating the coding process and looking at pragmatic functions in discourse needed to be the priority so that the analysis would allow for the exploration of the verbal communicative acts that emerged from the literature review. The Face-PCC analytical framework enabled me to examine the data for the presence of relevant PCC or potentially non-PCC acts in the particular context and to explore the relationship between the PCC elements and cultural factors.

The audio-recordings captured real-life contexts, as the participants did not have to place themselves in a totally different situation from their usual practice. Knowledge of the patients' backgrounds has provided the necessary contextualisation and has strengthened the interpretation of the language used in the consultations. The in-depth interviews with the doctors also played an important role. They provided clarification regarding (1) the extent to which Western communication practice is acquired during medical education and further professional experience, (2) the doctors' backgrounds and professional mindset and (3) an insight into the patients' perspectives. A commonly cited shortcoming of interviews is that they only provide anecdotal stories that are based on subjective experience; however, this aspect does not necessarily spoil the qualitative data. It rather added significant value to the findings. The physician participants' stories were extremely helpful to contextualise the details of the communication observed in the data.

8.10 Limitations of This Study

There are some limitations to this study. First, the small sample size of eight physician participants impacts on the generalisation of the findings regarding consultations strategies. All the doctors had engaged in practicing as physicians and had sufficient knowledge of communicating with older patients in the home settings. However, more nuanced findings may have been obtained with a wider pool of participants, representing a range of expertise and age or experience of interacting with older patients.

Furthermore, the findings from the consultation data are limited to the most personal setting – the patients' homes, where the professionals regularly visit the patient over months or years, and the patient offers tea or coffee to the professionals during or at the end of the consultation. Thus, the degree of formality or familiarity was largely influenced by personal relationships. The findings may be very different for consultations in hospital settings, for example.

The findings are also largely affected by the physicians' perspective. It would not have been possible to access the patient participants without the presence of the medical team, and no access could be secured beyond the consultations themselves. This means that I was not able to interview the patients and their family members as I had initially intended. This limitation came about because my observations were scheduled to fit in with the professionals' daily timetable, and we all travelled in the same car together to the patients' homes. Due to time constraints and availability, the timetable for their patients seemed less flexible. I could have considered alternative platforms to elicit Japanese patients' or family's perspectives: for example, using phone or email to ask questions and gain their responses, but this would have raised challenging practical and ethical issues. However, this might be achieved in a separate study, focusing on the patient perspectives.

All the data are naturally occurring data, and I intended to capture exactly what was said in each situation. If I had given myself some extra time to follow-up the specific utterances and their meanings with the doctor during the period of fieldwork, the issue would have been less significant. I would strongly recommend that the researcher secures access to a wide range of patients, allowing them to elicit the patients' opinions without the presence of the professionals.

8.11 Suggestions for Further Investigations

I have attempted to examine the concepts and theories of PCC, focusing on the exchanges between older adults and physicians in medical consultations. The findings reveal that the communicative acts are displayed by the professionals to a noticeable extent but that they are also shaped by culture-specific styles. Many elements of the PCC acts offer potential areas for future work.

First, the research protocol of this study employs multiple qualitative evidence, including observational fieldwork, field notes, audio recordings and qualitative interviewing, combined with the review of physical materials such as textbooks and manuals in the educational context. This methodological approach is one of the main contributions of this study, and it could be further extended to ensure that a researcher, by being in the field, cannot only observe but also identify further opportunities for data collection and monitor the quality of data collection. This does not necessarily mean prolonged periods of fieldwork but securing separate opportunities for attending relevant seminars or workshops would be extremely helpful to understanding the local setting and different healthcare situations and can potentially be another opportunity for collecting supplemental data.

In addition, the main data were audio-recordings of naturally occurring patient-professional interactions. Inevitably, ethical concerns were involved, which was the main reason why the analysis largely considers the participants' verbal acts through audio data, even though some cultures regard non-verbal elements as far more important. Further research could include in-depth investigation of non-verbal communication such as visual clues (i.e. facial expressions, handshakes, gestures), distance (personal space) and physical appearance by video recordings, and the arrangement of written texts (i.e. handwriting or font styles, the physical layout of a document or a web page).

The functional categorisation of the audio data was the key to analysing the discourse and finding the characteristics of the participants' speech acts. I processed transcribing, translating and categorising manually and focused only on clear examples in this manual process. This inevitably leaves room for errors. Working with at least one other researcher who checks interpretations would help reduce the margin for errors and, also, considering the analytical activity and useful tools in collaboration, would make the analytic process more efficient and avoid missing potential examples.

Not only face-to-face but also written communication between family members and multiple participants in different area of expertise (e.g. community and hospital doctors, dentists, nurses, therapists, carers, care home staff, care managers) was noticed in the fieldwork. The exploration of written communication could provide further insight into the application of PCC in a wide range of healthcare settings. During the fieldwork, I observed a variety of communication forms: the patients' families and carers keep handwritten notebooks to record the patient's physical and mental conditions, activities, meals, visitors, their observation, etc. Short-stay care homes also keep a record of the patient regarding the same information, for the purpose of transferring it to health professionals of the patient. Some medical teams and families keep a digital record about the same information above. Internal records between the professionals are also maintained, including their observation. This multiple written information is involved in any handover process in health, social care and home settings, particularly for the patient with dementia. In future research, the detailed investigation of written materials could shed further light on healthcare practices that may be conducive to PCC.

Finally, the mixed method I applied is one of the examples for various methodologies, and this can be transferable to other settings and different countries. The patient–doctor communication may vary depending on the situations, such as interactions in community clinics, hospital settings, telephone or online video consultations, or emergency care. Further investigation and evidence of PCC would certainly benefit many other specialists, patients and their families. Although it is assumed that the clinical communication models can improve the skillsets of doctors in the patient–doctor relationship, other factors such as the access, scope of treatment and transitions of care need to be considered. PCC skills training to young professionals and medical and nursing students would become a tool to encourage them to apply their human skills in their interactions with patients and help to reduce the negative effects from physical impairment and anxieties in their patients.

9 Appendices

9.1 A List of the Transcription Notation

The transcript notation used in this book was developed by Gail Jefferson (Hepburn & Bolden, 2013; Jefferson, 2004) and includes the following symbols.

Transcription Symbol	Referent
[	Left square bracket denotes a point where overlapping speech occurs.
]	Right square bracket indicates a point at which overlapping utterances end.
(.)	A full stop inside brackets denotes a micro pause but of no significant length.
(3.0)	A number inside brackets denotes a timed pause, represented in seconds.
.	The period indicates a falling or final, intonation.
,	A comma indicates 'continuing' intonation.
: :	Colons indicate the stretching of the sound just preceding them. The more the colons, the longer the stretching.
=	Continues utterance with no break or pause. One at the end of a line and another at the start of the next line or shortly thereafter.
-	A hyphen indicates a cut-off or self-interruption.
word	Underlining indicates stress or emphasis. The more the underlining, the greater the emphasis.
> <	Arrows surrounding the talk show that the pace of the speech has quickened.
< >	Arrows in this direction show that the pace of the speech has slowed down.
(( ))	Double brackets appear with a description of events by the transcriber.
(word)	When part of an utterance is in parentheses, this indicates uncertainty on the transcriber's part, but represents a likely possibility.
↑	When an upward arrow appears, it means that there is a rise in intonation.
↓	When a downward arrow appears, it means that there is a drop in intonation.
→	An arrow like this denotes a particular sentence of interest to the analyst.
hhh	Hearable aspiration may represent breathing, laughter, etc.
Hum(hh)our	A bracketed 'hh' means that there was laughter within the talk.
£	A smile voice – the speaker is smiling while speaking.

9.2 A Summary of Educational Materials Introducing Western Clinical Communication Models for Medical Education Use in Japan

MATERIAL TYPE	REFERENCE	THEORIES ADAPTED
Key textbooks introducing Western models for medical interviews written by Japanese authors	*Medical Interviews for Beginners* (Saito, 2000)	• The three-function approach to the medical interview (Cole & Bird, 1994) *(1) Gathering data to understand the patient's problems* *(2) Developing rapport* *(3) Education and motivation*
	Medical Interview: Evidence-based Approach (Mukohara, 2006)	• The Calgary-Cambridge Guide (Silverman *et al.*, 2013)
	Diagnostics[1] (Noguchi & Fukuhara, 2008)	• Macy Model of Doctor-Patient Communication (Kalet *et al.*, 2004)
Japanese translations of the original Western texts	*The Medical Interview: The Three-function Approach* (Cole & Bird, 1994)	• The three-function approach to the medical interview to communicate with patients, including basic interviewing skills and managing common challenging situations. In the latest third edition of the original literature, the three-function approach is amended: *Build the Relationship, Assess and Understand* and *Collaborative Management* (Cole & Bird, 2014).
	How to Break Bad News: A Guide for Health Care Professionals (Buckman, 2000)	• The six-step protocol is a set of guidelines in situations of delivering bad news; however, the guidelines also provide a model for effectively communicating less challenging information to patients as well, which are based on coherent and consistent principles of the guidelines.

9.3 Details of the Instances From the Face-PCC Analysis

FACE-PCC CATEGORY			INSTANCE of CASE	CASE NUMBER (CONSULTATIONS A)	CASE NUMBER (CONSULTATIONS B)
I. Attends to Patient's Positive Face 71/18 in total (PCC/non-PCC)	*a. Identifies issues that the patient wishes to address* 20/12 in total	1. INITIAL GENERAL REMARKS [GR]	11	9, 14	17, 19, 20, 21, 22, 24, 26, 27, 28
		2. GRADUALLY MOVES FROM OPEN TO CLOSED QUESTIONS [OtoC]	9	7, 9, 10	17, 19, 22, 24, 27, 28
		3. [Potentially non-PCC] SEQUENCE OF CLOSED QUESTIONS AT THE BEGINNING [SeC]	12	1, 2, 3, 4, 5, 12, 13	16, 18, 22, 23, 25
	b. Actively listens to the patient 20/4 in total	1. REPETITION, PARAPHRASING AND INTERPRETATION [Lis]	20	1, 2, 4, 7, 8, 9, 10, 11, 12, 14	15, 16, 17, 18, 19, 23, 24, 26, 27, 28
		2. [Potentially non-PCC] INTERRUPTION [Itr]	4	1, 3, 12	16
	c. Displays empathy and acceptance 31/2 in total	1. UNDERSTANDING AND APPRECIATION OF THE PATIENT'S FEELINGS [Und]	12	3, 4, 6, 8, 9, 10, 11, 14	19, 25, 26, 27
		2. EXPRESSIONS OF POSITIVE REGARD [PR]	15	1, 4, 6, 9, 10, 11, 12, 14	17, 18, 20, 24, 25, 26, 27
		3. SILENCE AS EMPATHIC ANTICIPATION [Sil]	4	14	17, 26, 27
		4. [Potentially non-PCC] BEING JUDGEMENTAL [Jud]	2	1, 8	0
II. Attends to Patient's Negative Face 51/7 in total (PCC/non-PCC)	*a. Works towards shared decision-making* 31/3 in total	1. SHARING UNDERSTANDING [SU]	13	3, 4, 7, 10, 11, 13	17, 18, 19, 22, 24, 27, 28
		2. SHARING THINKING [ST]	12	3, 4, 7, 14	16, 17, 18, 21, 22, 26, 27, 28
		3. OFFERING SUGGESTIONS [OS]	6	3, 4, 14	22, 27, 28
		4. [Potentially non-PCC] NO SHARED DISCUSSION [NoSD]	3	11, 17	22
	b. Leaves space for the patient 15/3 in total	1. OPEN QUESTIONS THAT OCCUR THROUGHOUT THE SESSION [OQ]	4	6, 9	17, 20
		2. CHECKING FOR UNDERSTANDING [CU]	11	1, 2, 3, 4, 8, 10	19, 20, 24, 27, 28
		3. [Potentially non-PCC] DIRECTIVES [Dir]	3	1, 4, 12	0
	c. Respects the patient's freedom 5/1 in total	1. LINGUISTIC DEFERENCE [LD]	5	2, 4, 9, 10	26
		2. [Potentially non-PCC] TOUCHING WITHOUT ASKING [TW]	1	0	1

9.4 Full Transcripts of All the Interviews With Physician Participants

The following section contains the interview transcripts with six physician participants. The transcripts are divided into small paragraphs, and the number at the beginning of each paragraph is used to be referred to in the main texts of the book.

Interview – D1

Researcher: Has your [communication] style [with patients] changed over the past 18 years?

18年間の中で、先生ご自身のスタイルが変わってきていますか。

1 I think it's constantly changing. I've always been shy and withdrawn, and I'm not good at talking in front of people. I feel very nervous when meeting someone for the first time and am not sociable; so, I've always wondered if I can communicate with patients well. I prefer to listen to other people. Even when talking with friends, I don't do well talking with many people at one time but prefer listening one-on-one.
それはもう常に変化していると思いますね。僕自身は、昔から引っ込み思案で恥ずかしがり屋。人前で喋るのは苦手。初対面の人とかはすごく緊張するし、社交的じゃないので、患者さんとのコミュニケーションもうまくできるかなっていうのは昔から思っていました。人の話を聞くというのは比較的好きで、友達と話していても、多人数と話すのは苦手なんだけれど、一対一で聞くのは結構好きなんですね。

2 When I became a resident doctor and started to be responsible for patients, I had some profoundly memorable ones. There was a lady who was hospitalised for a heart disease called unstable angina, and when she was discharged from the hospital, she said, 'You truly listened to me. There are no other doctors like you'. I was moved and felt that I should keep that attitude going forward. At the same time, feelings of failure because my communication did not go well were my most common experience as a resident doctor.
研修医になって患者さんを担当した時に、思い出深い人も中にはいます。不安性狭心症という心臓の病気で入院したおばさんがいたんですけど、その人が退院する時に「先生は本当によく話を聞いてくれて、なかなか他にいない先生ですね」と言ってくれたんです。それが心に残って、そういう姿勢を大事にして行こうと思いました。一方で、コミュニケーションがうまくいかないから失敗したなという経験も研修医の時が一番多いです。

3 I was in charge of a patient with cerebral infarction. In general, these patients all vary regarding how severe the damage is and how much aftereffects remain. So, the patient and his family were very anxious.

I was in the second year of my residency, and I had to explain to the patient's wife by myself. I thought I tried my best, but she got even more worried about the situation. It became an issue, and I had to bring the head of the neurology department in to explain to the patient's wife and son again. Thinking about it now, it was because of the unfortunate way [subtle difference] I had spoken. I should have spoken accurately but without causing anxiety in the listener. There are situations where a resident doctor should not be left to talk to a particular patient [or family] alone, which I know about now but didn't know at that time.
脳梗塞の患者さんがいて、どのくらいのダメージなのか、後遺症がどのくらい残るのかとかは千差万別なので、患者も家族もすごく不安なんです。僕が研修医2年目のとき、僕一人でその患者さんの奥さんに説明をしました。僕は一生懸命説明したつもりだったんですけど、奥さんがそれで一層不安に思ってしまって。息子さんと神経内科の部長を含めてまたもう一度説明しないといけない事態になったんですね。今考えると、微妙な話し方のせいなんです。正確なことを話しつつも、不安を持たせない話し方っていうのもある。この患者さんには、研修医一人にさせてはまずいとか、今だったらわかるんですけれど、当時は分からない。

4 I finally felt like I really learned communication skills when I started my ninth year of training as a family physician. It felt like the emphasis it places on communication skills opened my eyes. Looking back now, I think what you learn in the first few years is really integral, and whether you can learn basic communication skills in the first few years as a resident doctor will affect you much later. Unfortunately, I had no opportunity to take a formal class on the subject, and as a result, I ran into difficulties in real-life experience [due to insufficient knowledge of the skills].
コミュニケーションについてしっかり学んだなって思えたのは、家庭医療の研修に9年目から入ったんですけど、それはかなりコミュニケーションのスキルを重視するので、そこで目から鱗のような感じでした。こうやって振り返ってみると最初の数年間での学びというのはすごく大きくて、研修医になって最初の数年間のうちにしっかりと基礎的なスキルを学べるかがあとまで響くと思います。僕は残念ながらコミュニケーションのフォーマルな授業は受けなかったけれども、それで実際に困ったという経験が沢山ありました。

5 Unfortunately, I had no opportunity to take a formal class on the subject, and I experienced many real-life difficulties as a result. I don't think it's a good thing. Mentors may give feedback on examination practices, but I think it's quite rare that they give regular feedback on how to communicate with patients in the field. I think, ideally, it would be better if mentors gave real advice like 'don't you think it

would have been better if you had talked to them like this?' or 'interacting with them like this works well'.
僕は残念ながらコミュニケーションのフォーマルな授業は受けなかったけれども、それで実際に困ったなあという経験が沢山ありました。それはあまり良くないと思うんですね。診療のプラクティスに関しては指導医がフォードバックしてくれるけれど、コミュニケーションの取り方に関して現場でこう指導医がちゃんとフィードバックしてくれるっていうのは意外に少ないなと思っていて。本来はもうちょっとそこも指導医がいて、そこはこういう風に話した方がよかったんじゃないかとか、こういう接し方だとうまくいくよっていうのを本当は指導してくれると、もっといいと思うんですけどね。

R: When you were a medical student, were there lectures about interviewing patients?
先生の学部時代に患者さんとの問診のレクチャーはありましたか。

6 I was in medical school from 1994 to 2000. At that time, there was no communication skills training and simulated patients had not yet been introduced in education. So, I have hardly any memories of being taught about the subject. There was training on clinical diagnostic practice and that left a huge impression on me. The normal lectures were about diseases, but this class had interactive small group sessions with the professor. They explained that, if a patient comes like this, you need to ask like this and conduct a physical exam. I really enjoyed it.
僕の時代は、1994年から2000年の6年間だったんですけど、コミュニケーション実習がない時代だったので、模擬患者さんもまだ教育に入ってきていない時代で、コミュニケーションの教育を受けたと言う記憶がほとんどないです。臨床診断学実習というのはありました。それがすごく記憶に残っていて、普通のレクチャーは病気についてのものですけど、それは小グループで先生のインタラクティブな、患者さんがこういう風にきたらこういう風に聞いて、体を触診して診察するんだよみたいな話を聞けたので、僕はそれがすごく好きだったんですね。

7 There was one geriatrics lecture that left a huge impression on me. The professor was more of a generalist, so I think their stance was closer to that of a family doctor or general practitioner. They taught me how to listen to heart sounds. [...] During the rotation, I was told to go take the history of an older man with dementia who had been admitted. Even though I was only a student, I went to his bedside. I greeted him and introduced myself. He started to make a scene, shouting, 'this guy is an alien', 'an alien came'. I was really nervous and also quite shocked, because I didn't know much about dementia.
すごく印象に残っているのは老年病学ジェリアトリックスで、先生はジェネラリストなので、家庭医とか総合診療医に近いスタンスだったと思うんですけど。胸の聴診の聞き方を教えてくれたんですね。[...] そのローテーションの頃、認知症のおじいちゃんが入院してる時に問診してこいと言われて、学生だけで、そのおじいちゃんのベッドサイドに行きました。挨拶と自己紹介をしました。そのおじいちゃんが、こいつは宇宙人だ、宇宙人が来たって騒ぎ始めたんですね。こっちもすごく緊張していたし、認知症がこういう症状でとかはあまり知らなかったので、かなりショックを受けました。

8 I am not saying he discriminated against me but being treated that way made me feel desolate. After that, the geriatrics professor followed up with me and told me that things like this happen. In those days, there was no training on how to communicate as there is now. We were just thrown in front of patients and told to listen to them. That's why incidents like that happened. So, I think it's very important to follow-up after such experiences, to reflect and think about why it happened. Even experiences you feel are negative can lead to huge growth.
差別とまでは言わないけどそう扱われて、寂しい思いになったんですけどね。そのあとに、老年病の先生が、まあそういうこともあるよってフォローしてくれました。今みたいに、こういう風にコミュニケーションを取りましょうというトレーニングは当時全くなかったんですけど、いきなり患者さんの前にボンと出される訳ですよね、はい患者さんの話聞いてって。だからそういうプチ事件が起こりますよね。だからそのあとのフォローがすごく大事だと思っていて、リフレクションとか、なぜこういう風になったんだろうねというのを全部、ネガティブに思った体験でも、すごく強い学びに繋がります。

R: I happened to think of this during fieldwork, but I was wondering who has the right to speak freely at your clinic…
フィールドワーク中に気になったのですが、クリニックの中で発言権を持っている方というのは…

9 In the clinic, it's the most experienced nurse, rather than the chief nurse. The previous chief was a very powerful person, but the experienced nurses could speak their minds even to them. She [the experienced nurse] also seem to admonish the residents, and I sometimes thought that might seem wrong from the perspective of the nurses. Some nurses guess right through their intuition. If the nurse and the doctor had a relationship where the nurse could admonish the doctor more directly in that case, it would be great. On the other hand, there are many institutions where a nurse cannot say anything. Some institutions allow nurses to tell the doctor afterward that 'the way you spoke was not good, doctor' if the nurses notice something bad, but others do not. I think more institutions have a culture that forbids it, though. Also, there are cases where the doctor is aware of his or her authority and can communicate humbly. Being humble is not necessary,

but if they have more conversation [with staff] on a daily basis, such exchanges may come naturally.
クリニックの中では、師長さんじゃなく、ベテランの看護師さん。前の師長さんは結構力のある人だったんですが、その人に対しても発言できるのがそのベテランの看護師さんなんですね。研修医とかにも諭すような感じで、看護師から見て、これ違うんじゃないかなって思うことってあるんですよね。看護師の直感が当たっていることもあるので、そういう時に直接的に諭すような感じで言える、そういう関係性が医師と看護師の間にあるといいですね。その一方で言えないという組織もいっぱいある。あのドクターのこういうところがダメだって気付いて、後で看護師が「先生あの言い方はちょっと」って言える組織と言えない組織とある。言えない方が多いかもしれないですね。ドクター自身が自分の権威を意識してあえてへりくだるような形でコミュニケーションを取れるかっていうのもある。へりくだるまでいかなくても日常的に会話が多ければ、その中で自然に言えることもある。

R: I heard before that only about 20% of nurses in Japan are male.
先ほど男性の看護師さんの割合は日本では2割と聞きました。

10 There are not many. Although there are more in psychiatry. There are more male nurses in psychiatry because they need to be able to firmly hold patients. In contrast, there are few in clinics. Hospital wards also have many male nurses.
少ないですよ。精神科に多いですけど。患者さんをガシッと捕まえないといけないので、男性看護師が多いんですよ精神科は。クリニックとかは少なくて。病院の入院病棟にも男性看護師は多いですね。

R: Research on gender differences has shown that female doctors spend more time with patients, are more empathetic and explain things better.
ジェンダーに関する研究結果で、女性医師の方がより長い時間患者と過ごして、より共感的でよく説明すると言われています。

11 Female doctors spend longer with patients, even outpatients, around the world, and they also tend to have higher empathy scores. While some of the difference may be innate, women have stronger skills for providing care. The same is true for everyday communication. Perhaps male communication is more goal-oriented than empathetic, while women talk to each other for the sake of empathising. I think everyday communication has a considerable influence on [caring].
世界的に外来でも女性の方が［時間が］長いっていうのがあって、共感スコアも女性の方がだいたい高いんですよね。そこのジェンダー差っていうのは、生まれつきのものもあるかもしれないですけど、女性の場合はケアする力が強いですね。日常的なコミュニケーションもそうですよね。男性のコミュニケーションは共感よりも目的志向というか。女性同士は共感を求めて会話しますよね。日常的なコミュニケーションもかなり影響してると思うので。

R: During my most recent fieldwork, I often heard patients talk about their mental pain and spiritual topics, and I feel how difficult it is for doctors.
今回のフィールドワーク中、 患者さんの心の痛み、スピリチュアルな発言を聞くことも多く、先生の大変さを常々感じます。

12 When I see older patients, I often hear the phrase 'I want to die' and think how I should respond to the statement, because you cannot show no reaction. If you do not say anything and leave without changing your facial expression, you are a robot. If you are told 'I want to die, doctor', you will be moved because you are a human, and the one who has to think of a response is the medical worker. This is not taught in medical school. This matter tests our powers of humanity and communication skills.
高齢者の方を見ていると、よく死にたいという言葉を聞くので、そこにどう答えていくかという。それを言われた時に、レスポンスゼロというわけにはいかないので。もし何も言わないで、何も表情一つ変えずに帰ってしまったら、ロボットですよね。人間だから絶対、死にたいと言われたら心を動かされるし、何か答えなきゃと思うのが医療従事者。そこは学校で教わらないこと。そこは自分の人間力とか、コミュニケーション力が問われるとは思います。

13 The other day, in a class for fourth-year students, I had a patient give a talk about her experience being ill. She has chronic kidney disease and has been on dialysis for 23 years. She started her presentation with an excellent first slide. 'Please find the area of this triangle. You all know how to do that, right? Now, please answer the next question. A patient says to you, "Doctor, please save me. Please save my life". Alright, what's your answer? It's difficult, isn't it? This is what medical care is about.' Then she started telling her story. I was very impressed by that introduction. It drove home that problems that you cannot answer will hit you one after another. Because medical students are only asked questions that have answers. They're better than anyone at solving quiz questions, but her point was whether they could answer a question like that.
先日4年生の学生に向けてある患者さんに闘病体験を話してもらったんですね。そのかたが慢性腎臓病のかたで、23年間も血液透析をやってる方なんですけど、すごくいいスライドを最初出されたんですね。1枚目のスライドが、この三角形の面積を求めてください。これみなさんわかりますよね。では、次の問題に答えてください。患者さんが、あなたにこう言いました。「先生、助けてください。私の命を助けてください。」はい、答えはなんですか。難しいですよね。医療というのはこういうものです。ここから話が始まって、いい掴みだって感動しました。答えないのない問題が現実ではボンボン降ってくるよっていう。医学生って答えのある問題ばかり解いてきてるから。クイズとか問題を解くのは誰よりも早いんだけれど、この問題に答えられるかっていう話ね。

14 With regard to communication skills, I think that we can now teach students the minimum level needed. Next, I think it will be important to teach compassion and empathy, although I feel this is still difficult. To do so, I think it will be crucial to teach students to listen to patient narratives and to intuit and think about how best to interact with the patient at that time. As an educator, I would like to tackle this challenge.
コミュニケーションスキルは、最低限のスキルは今は教えられるようになって、その次はコンパッションとかエンパシーの教育が重要になってくるんだと思う、まだ難しいところだと思いますけど。そういう時に患者さんのナラティブを聞いて、学生がきちんとこういう時にどう患者さんと接したらいいんだろうって感じたり考えたりする教育が大事かなと思っていて。そういうところを教育者としてはやっていきたいなと思っていますね。

R: Has your perspective changed since becoming an educator?
教育者になられたあとで、また意識は変わりましたか。

15 Since I have to teach students, I need to be a role model to some extent, so things like my professionalism have gone up. Also, the perspective of doing everything you can for the patient in front of you when practicing. After becoming an educator, I had to think about how best to convey that to a diverse group of students. If there is a student who can't do it well, what can I do to get them to learn it? In education, that sort of perspective comes in. There are several communication models, and I have found that it's important to teach them in a way that's easy to understand. There have been perspective changes like this.
学生に教えなきゃいけないので、自分が模範にある程度ならないといけないなっていう、プロフェッショナリズム的なものが少しだけ高まりました。あと現場にいるときは目の前の患者さんにベストを尽くすっていう視点ですよね。教育者になったあとは、それをどういう風に色んな人に伝えて学んでもらうかっていう視点があって、うまくできない人がいたとしたら、そういう人に学んでもらうとしたらどうしたらいいか。教育だとそういう視点が入ってきて、コミュニケーションのモデルというのがいくつかあって、そういうのをわかりやすく伝えていくっていうのも大事なんだなっていうことがわかりました。こうした視点の違いはありますね。

16 When I was working five or six days straight, I fully applied myself there and was not at all flexible. I now have some more emotional

leeway. Although practicing doctors are required to have a surprising amount of creativity to respond when a patient says 'I want to die', how they practice is in some ways limited. They must follow guidelines and evidence and can't stray from such things.
現場に週5日、6日、張り付いていたときはすごくそこに適用するのでなかなか余裕がないです。今は少し心の余裕が生まれているのもあるんですけど。意外と現場の医者は、患者に「死にたい」と言われた時のクリエイティビティは求められるけれども、医師としてのプラクティスのやり方はある程度縛りがあって、ガイドラインにしたがってとか、エビデンスにしたがってとか、そこから離れられないしとか。

17 I think that education should be more free. Education becomes boring as it becomes more rigid. In that sense, changing my position to that of an educator has changed my perspective toward freedom and creativity. I would like to use works of art [such as files and novels] when teaching empathy; otherwise, students will find it uninteresting or too rigid. It is better to cultivate the students' sensitivities through artworks and listening to real patients' stories.
教育っていうのはもっと自由であっていいと思っていて、教育は硬直化するほどつまらないものになっていくので、そういう意味では教育者に立場が変わったことでさらに自由さというか、クリエイティブにやった方がいいなと思っています。共感を教える時にアートを使ったりしていかないと学生もつまらないし窮屈だと思うんです。アートに触れたり患者さんの話を聞く中で感性を耕していく方がいいと思うんですね。

Interview – D2

Researcher: Do you think the style in which you communicate [with patients] has changed since you graduated from medical school?
医学部を卒業されてから、コミュニケーションスタイルが変わってきたと思いますか。

1 I don't think it has changed. Roughly speaking, the basics are the same. From my student days I did think of communication with outpatients, knowing how to treat them and such, as something that's just the way it is. So I did sometimes participate in some seminars about it on my own. So, on a general level, those superficial skills, such as active listening attentively, starting with an open question, or listening to the patient for three minutes – those haven't changed.
多分変わってないと思います。大雑把に言うと、素のものには変わりはないんです。ただ接遇スキルとかそういうのも含めたコミュニケーションの、外来でのね、僕は学生の時から「そういうものだ」と思っていて、自分からそういう独自のセミナーみたいなのに時々参加してたんです。それで、いわゆる一般的なレベルのこと、表面上のスキルですね、傾聴するとか、オープンクエスチョンで始めるとか3分間聞いてみたいな、ああいうところはあまり変わりないんです。

2 There are some things I have naturally, for example, the ability to make small talk, which hasn't changed in me. I guess it depends on your definition of 'the style in which I communicate'. As I've gained experience, there are some advanced skills that I've acquired later, such as in breaking bad news, and listening to multiple people at the same time. If you call those changes, then there has been some change. But my 'style' has not changed.
ただ雑談をしたりって持って生まれたものがありますよね、そこは変わりないです。コミュニケーションスタイルの定義によると思うんですけど。ただ経験を積むにつれてバッドニュースの告知とか、複数の人を同時に聞くとか、ちょっとアドバンスなタイプのスキルっていうのは後から会得したものですね。そこが変わったといえば変わったんですけど、スタイルに変わりはないです。

R: Do you think that individual differences [amongst young doctors] is something that further develops after leaving medical school?
医学部をでたあとは個人差というのは広がってくるものですか。

3 I think it is. The biggest difference is whether or not you get feedback and whether you get an opportunity to reflect, especially when you are young. Once you get to a certain point, no one ends up saying anything. There's a big difference depending on whether or not there is feedback about something that went well or didn't go well. Fortunately, I did do this sort of communication skills training, so I had plenty of opportunities to see how many people did things, for feedback, and to reflect on my own practices too.
広がってくると思います。一番の差はフィードバックがあるかどうかですよね。自分で振り返る場面があるかどうか。得に若いときは。ある程度までいくと誰も何も言わなくなりますけど。うまくいったこといかなかったことフィードバックがあるかどうかで、だいぶ違ってくると思うんです。僕は幸いにして、こういうコミュニケーショントレーニングをしていましたので、あと人勢の人たちのスタイルのもみて、フィードバックをかけながら自分のも振り返ったりする機会に恵まれていました。

4 [Here in Japan], many doctors in our generation have no opportunity to receive feedback. Young doctors who graduated within the past 10 years have better opportunities of feedback compared to our generation before 2000, who had none. Even more so, in our generation, there was absolutely nothing. [In the worst case], if you are in private practice, you may risk losing customers [patients]. In hospitals, unless a lot of patient complaints are made against you, your communication style as a doctor does not affect your salary. This is not just about

doctors. In the graduate school I went to in the US, students would leave the classroom if the lecturer's performance was bad. The lecturer won't be chosen to teach for the next semester if his or her lectures are dull, no matter how excellent his or her achievements are. But this does not happen in Japan.
多くの医師たちは全くフィードバックの機会がないです。若い先生達、卒後10年くらいの先生たちは、昔に比べればフィードバックの機会は多少なりともあるけど、2000年以前に卒業した人というのは全くないです。まして我々世代はゼロです。開業医ではお客さん来なくなるっていうのがありますけど、病院ではクレームがいっぱい来たら別ですけど、そうでもなければ、別にそれで給料が上がったり下がったりしない。医師に限ったことではないですけど、アメリカの僕がいた大学院では、先生の授業がつまらなければみんな帰りますよ。で、次のセメスターで採用されないですよ。どんなに優れた業績があっても、つまらない話されたらね。日本ではこういうのないですから。

5 Only the surface level of the concept 'empathic communication' is becoming prevalent. It's tested in the OSCE, so all students are thinking from the very beginning about where to put empathic statements in an interview, because they will lose marks if they don't appear empathetic. But there is no evidence. There is no evidence [in Japan] on whether the patients truly feel persuaded or satisfied with empathic remarks. In Japan, communication is a 'ritual form' like the tea ceremony, flower arranging, judo, karate and so on. When it comes to talking about its hidden aspects, it becomes more religious.
共感的コミュニケーションと言われるものが一人歩きをしていって、学生達はOSCEの試験で出るので共感的態度を言葉を示さないと点が下がるんです。学生は皆、どこで共感的発言を入れようか最初から考えているんです。でもエビデンスがないんですよ。本当に共感的な発言をすると患者さんが納得するのか満足するのかどうかエビデンスがないんです。日本は、コミュニケーションは「道」ですから。茶道、花道、柔道、空手とか、型ですから。見えないところの説明になると宗教的になるんです。

R: Some earlier research papers say that Japanese doctors seem to be very cold.
過去の研究論文で、日本人医師はとても冷たいという一説があります。

6 Americans praise their children so much, you know, saying 'My kid is the best'. Those who look critically at us, Japanese people say that Japanese parents do not praise their children or nurture their self-esteem. Certainly, there are cultural differences and, let's say, cultural relativism. We don't hug each other every time we meet in Japan, do we? The number of international workers has increased in Tokyo in

the past 10 years, and the way of thinking has diversified. It's been changing, noticeably when giving bad news. Until about my fifth year as a fully-fledged doctor after finishing as a resident, delivering bad news to cancer patients was never an option in Japan.
めちゃくちゃ褒めるじゃないですかアメリカ人は、オーバーにうちの子供はナンバーワンだって。批判的に見る人は、日本人の親は子供を褒めないし自尊心を育てないと言う。文化相対性主義もありますけどやはり違いはあると思います。日本では会うたびにハグする文化はないです。ここ10年東京では外国人が増えて、考え方も多様になっていますし、とくに変わったのは告知のところです。僕が研修医から医師になって5年目くらいまではがんの人に告知するなんてなかったです。

7 Now, we do almost 100% of the time. However, there are some traditions left, such as informing family members of it without the patient's agreement. Which is illegal in the United States. Some students come here [to the clinic] regularly, and they may even do some sessions themselves, sometimes taking videos themselves. We have quite a lot of opportunity to use those videos, for instance, for reflection.
今は、ほぼ100%します。ただ本人の同意を得ないで家族に話すとか、そういうところは今も残っています。アメリカでは違法ですけどね。定期的に学生さんがここに来たり、自分でもセッションをしたりして、たまに自分でビデオ撮るんですよ。そのビデオを見せながらやったり、機会が結構あるので、その都度、反省をする機会はあります。

R: What sort of reflection?
どんな反省ですか。

8 My father also used to be a doctor, and he had this specific 'doctor tone'. In everyday life, he was just an ordinary guy. But once he was at work, he'd talked in this certain tone, talking as if to say, 'I know everything about you'. So, there's this sort of 'doctor tone'. That is something I don't like. And I sense when we're adopting it.
うちの父も医者をしていたので、医者口調ってあるんですよ。普通に生活してるときは大した人間じゃないんですよ。仕事場にいくと、あたかも私はあなたのことをよく知ってますよみたいな雰囲気で話をしたり、そういう医者口調ってあるんです。その医者口調になってる、それが僕すごく嫌なんですよ。それになってるなっていうのは感じるんです。

9 He [the doctor in the video] doesn't listen, doesn't say 'it's okay', doesn't answer. The way he speaks to patients and staff differs. He doesn't apologise for keeping the patient waiting. He's somewhat arrogant. The patient is mystified by the doctor's words. My father was doing this too. A nice impression but true feelings are left unsaid. Doctors have to say something even when they don't know whether it's okay or not. So, they say, we shall see. If the patient asks 'Will it

get better?', they say 'Let's hope so'. And if you're not careful this can come out in your daily life too.
聞かない。結論言わない。大丈夫って言わない。答えない。患者に対する言い方とスタッフに対する言い方が違う。待たせたことについて謝らない。なんとなく偉いんです。煙に巻こうとしている。うちの父もこんな感じ。優しそうな感じなんですけど本音は言えてない。大丈夫かどうか、わからなくても医者は何か言わないといけない。困るので、様子みましょうとか。治るんですかって言われたら、いや治るといいですねとか。下手すると日常生活にも出てくるので。

10 Everyone says 'patient-centred', but I haven't felt I can fit in the concept of patient-centredness. I don't think anyone can be centred in medical care. I don't think anything can be centred in it. It is difficult to know what to say to a patient who is in a really difficult situation, without learning through experience. In the articles I gave you, there's an episode I wrote about 15 years ago, which is about how to answer questions from patients in difficult situations. There is no answer. Well, there is an answer. You will ask why he or she thinks so and show empathy with the feelings. But this is only superficial. There is a huge difference between those who can find the right words to say and those who cannot as medical professionals, as people who provide care.
患者中心って言いながら、僕は患者中心っていう考え方そのものが、ちょっとまだ違和感があるんです。誰が中心のものでもないと思うんです医療っていうのは。どこが中心でもないんじゃないかと思うんですけど。本当に辛い状況にいる患者さんに対して何を言うかは、場数を踏まないとどう声を掛けるかって難しい。差し上げた資料の中に、15年前に書いたエピソードが入ってるんですけど、辛い状況にいる患者さんからの質問になにを答えるかっていう。まあ答えなんかないですよ。一応ありますよ、なんでそう思ったのかを聞いて気持ちに対して共感してとか。でもそんなのは通り一遍のことで。そこでちゃんとした言葉がかけられる人とかけられない人で、医者として、ケアをする者としてだいぶ違いがあるじゃないですか。

11 For health professionals, especially for young doctors, what you consider in those contexts isn't something technical but, rather, how to handle feelings. There are our experiences, narratives, the environments we were raised in. So, it is important to talk to the patient bearing in mind such factors. To some extent, it is partly based in skill and partly not. I stopped writing about teaching communication skills for a reason like this, because there were so many requests for 'tips' on how to communicate well.
プロとしては、とくに若い先生は、そう言う場面になったらどう考えるかっていうのは気持ちの持ち方であって、そこはテクニックじゃないと。それは場数もあるし、ナラティブもあるし、育ってきた環境もあるから、そういうのを踏まえた声かけが大事です。ある程度、スキルとスキルでない部分があるので。途中でコミュニケーションのことを書くのをやめたというのはそれに近くて、依頼がすごく多くて、こうするととてもうまいコミュニケーションができるみたいなのを皆求めていたんです。

Interview – D3

Researcher: Do you think the style in which you communicate [with patients] has changed since you graduated from a medical school?
医学部を卒業されてから、コミュニケーションスタイルが変わってきたと思いますか。

1 That is a difficult question. I think it's changed, but what's changed? There might be several things. The first one is that, as I just told you, fundamentally I don't construct relationships in which it has to be me that's the doctor (in charge). For example, when I was a medical student, I knew that [students] are seen as unreliable by patients, so I wanted to have patients come to rely on me, even just a little bit. So I made an effort to build a good relationship with the patient, as much as possible.
それは難しい質問ですね。変わってるとは思うんですけど、何が変わってきているか。いくつかあるかもしれません。一つは [担当医が] 私じゃなければいけないっていう関係作りは基本的にしないってお話をさっきしましたけど、例えば、医学生の頃とか、患者さんからすると全く頼りにならない存在だったりするので、少しでも患者さんに自分を頼りにしてほしいっていうので最大限その患者さんとの関係が良く構築されるように努力しました。

2 From the perspective of continuously maintaining quality of care, even when it's me that's a whole family's doctor, I still make sure that I don't create a relationship that would need to involve me. No matter which doctor comes in, it's fine. As long as they're seen by a GP, or they ask staff at this clinic, they'll be fine. This is the kind of relationship I build every time.
継続的に、ケアの質を保つという観点からすると、私が一家庭医として関わる場合でも、私じゃなきゃダメっていう関係性を作らないようにする。どの医師が来ても、少なくとも家庭医が見れば大丈夫だ、もしくはこの診療所のスタッフにお願いすれば大丈夫だっていう関係性を患者さんときちんと構築していく。

3 I have worked here relatively long, but doctors do often change workplace for training and such. Even if a patient really likes a certain doctor, it is unlikely that the doctor can be involved from one patient's birth to death. 'Taking over' [from one doctor to another] is just unavoidable. We even do group practice, where

multiple people are involved. That sort of style is more... I think what's changed is a focus towards building a relationship in order to maintain quality of care, but not to make it so that only I can understand the patient.
僕は比較的長くいますけど、研修とかで職場を変えることが多いんですよね。この先生がすごくいいってお話があったとしても、その患者さんが生まれてから死ぬまで一人のお医者さんが関われるかっていうと [医師の存在は] すごく断片的なんですよね。どうしても引き継ぎは必要で、グループプラクティスといって複数で関わったりもするので、そういったスタイルが比較的、ケアの質を保つためにも関係性を作るけれども、自分とじゃないと話が通じないっていう関係性にしないようにコントロールするところに、変わってきていると思います。

4 A resident doctor may see the patient, so the patient feels they can say they want to talk to an experienced doctor instead, it's very difficult to train the residents. If patients say they'd have preferred [another specific] doctor, even if the resident did perform well, for them it's still not a success, is it? I would explain that any doctor can handle the fundamentals and that this resident may even listen to you better than me, things like that. Thus, since becoming a doctor, I reckon there's been a change, both from the perspective of a supervisor and as a family doctor, from building a relationship just with yourself, towards this current style.
研修医が行くこともあるので、ベテランのお医者さんがいいって患者さんが当然のように言う関係性になってしまうとね、研修医としてはすごく研修しにくいんです。患者さんが「[あの] 先生がよかったな」って言うとね、研修医としては、研修医のパフォーマンスが良かったとしても、うまくいかないですよね。どの医師でも基本的なことは対応しますし、私よりも研修医の方がよく話を聞いてくれるかもしれませんよ、みたいな形で、指導者っていう観点からも、一家庭医としての観点からも、自分だけと関係性を作るってスタイルからは今のようなスタイルに医者になってから変わってきている部分だと思います。

R: Becoming the chief of the clinic was the major factor?
所長になられた部分が大きいんでしょうか。

5 Yes, it is, and becoming a supervising doctor is also a large factor. I need to prepare an environment where younger doctors can train properly. I think these elements certainly have an influence. Another thing is, while the core basics haven't changed, I have had opportunities to learn more technical, finer-detailed methods over the years; I do think things have become more technical. I have changed how I respond while listening to the patient's story, especially whether to let something pass without comment, whether to remain silent, when to add empathetic phrases and so on, but these

changes were only in minor or insignificant details. These are certain skills to build a better relationship with patients, in order to draw them towards us [health professionals] emotionally, or to remove as much anxiety as possible.
所長もそうだし、指導医になったという部分も大きいと思います。より後輩のドクター達がきちんと研修できる環境を整える。そういったところはあるんじゃないかなと思いますね。あと思いつくところで、もう一点、根本は変わってないんですけど、技術的な細かいテクニカルな技法とかは、年数を経るごとに学んだりする機会があって、テクニカルなことは増やしていると思います。話を聞きながらどういう風に返答するか、流すか、沈黙をとるかとか、どのタイミングで共感的なフレーズを入れてみるかとかそういうところは変わってきたと思いますけど、枝葉が変わったという感じです。より効果的に関係性を作るために、患者さんの気持ちをこちら側に誘導するため、もしくは不安を取り除くためにです。

R: Was there any subject related to communication skills training when you were a medical student?
大学の中でコミュニケーション教育の関連した科目とかはありましたか。

6 I learnt about communication and such mostly after becoming a doctor. I learnt the content that should be ideally included in medical education after I became a resident doctor, although we could categorise that trainee period as being part of a student's education. At the end of my trainee period, I was participating in workshops on my own, and those experience became the basis of my skills. I don't think there's anything there that I was taught at the university.
コミュニケーションとかそういうことは、ほとんどは医者になってから教わりました。本来、医学教育に含まれるべきコンテンツを研修医になってから教わりました。学生教育の範疇といえば範疇ですけど。高学年の最後の方は自分でワークショップに参加するとか、そういうのが自分の基礎的な部分になっていると思います。大学の中で教わったってことはないかなと思う。

R: Did you have any role models?
お手本見みたいな方がいらっしゃったんですか。

7 No. I don't think I did. There was no textbook [on communication skills] back then, although there might be some now. After I graduated and became a doctor, though, I had contact with a lecturer in communication studies in the field of family medicine, and I had the opportunity to learn from them, for instance.
ない。なかったと思いますね。テキストもとくになかった、今はあるかもしれないけど僕の時はなかった。卒業して医者になってから、家庭医療の業界の中でコミュニケーション学の先生とかと接点ができて、教えてもらう機会とかは出てきましたけど。

8 As a child, I just knew I wanted to become a doctor, and what I was imagining back then was a normal doctor in a town. I thought I'd just like to be helpful to people, I wouldn't even mind going to a remote regional area, or maybe I could get involved in healthcare internationally, something like that. I had a naive childish notion of wanting to do some kind of work to help people in need.
子供の頃になんとなく医者になりたいと思ったんですけど、その時にイメージしていたのは普通に町にいる医者で、人の役に立てたらそれでいいかなとか、へき地に行ってもいいかなとか、国際保健とかに携わってもいいかなとかなんとなく困っている人の役に立つ仕事がしたいみたいに子供心に思っていました。

9 Family physicians and GPs do normally receive training in communication skills, but if we look at how things are currently in Japan, specialist doctors mostly don't learn these things when they're students, and even when they're residents – it's just straight-talking; there's little opportunity to learn about how to communicate. There are some people who can do it well naturally without receiving any training, and yes, they are wonderful. But, I think that it's important for education to raise the bottom line (i.e. improve the minimum quality), and it is not ideal that some doctors are good and some are not.
家庭医やGPはコミュニケーションに関するトレーニングをしていることが多いんですが、一般に日本の現状だと、スペシャリストになっている方達はほとんど学生時代に教わらず、研修でもストレートにこう言って、コミュニケーションを学ぶ機会も少ないと思います。中にはトレーニングを受けなくてもきちんとできる人っていうのもいて、そういう人達は素晴らしいって言われて、でも本来、教育って最低ライン、ボトムラインをあげることが重要なので、 医師によって当たり外れが大きいのはちょっとと思います。

R: Have you ever felt that communication is difficult with resident doctors when they come here?
研修医が先生のところに来て、コミュニケーションできてないなって感じることはありますか。

10 Yes, I have. But I can only provide technical support. If a doctor is not willing to communicate or looks down on patients – if they have fundamental issues like this, with their attitudes and values – it is very difficult for me to make any corrections there, because they're already grown up as an adult.
ありますよ。でも僕にできるのは、技術的な支援だけなんですよね。コミュニケーションする気がない人とか、患者さんを見下しているとか、そういう価値観とか根幹の問題を抱えている場合は、ほとんどの場合、修正は難しいですね。大人として出来上がっているので。

11 I can give some technical advice, or suggest they summarise what the person has said first, for instance. But personality-related issues are almost impossible to correct. However, sometimes it's not a problem with the learner, it's just a misdirection of effort. In that case, we'll talk about a range of things, and I'll give advice by suggesting how it might look to someone else, and how they might see it differently if they change such-and-such.
例えばこういうタイミングで、相手が言ったことをサマライズして話してみるといいとかテクニカルなアドバイスは言えるけれど、人間性に問題があるとなると修正はほぼ難しいですね。でも学習者だけの問題じゃなくて、本人の努力の方向性が違うだけだったりとか、その場合は色々話をしていく中で、他の人にはこう見えたりもするけど、こう変えてみると見え方が変わると思うとアドバイスするとか。

R: Your consultations included repetition and summaries at regular intervals. So, it was easy for us listening to understand what you were talking about. I felt that everyone in the same room understood what was going on.
先生のコンサルテーションは、リピートとサマライズを等間隔で入れてくださるので、聞いてるこちらがわかりやすい。その場にいる全員がわかりやすい空気を作ってくださっているなって感じました。

12 If you're not repeating or paraphrasing, it's easy to often misread someone's intentions. Japanese people especially tend to smile and sidestep things. The man we first met today is hard of hearing, and probably he didn't hear what I said. But I think he thought that it would be rude if he asked me to repeat what was said in that situation, so he just nodded and said 'yes, yes'. I can check if I have misheard what the person has said, but it's difficult to check about what I have said, unless I consciously confirm it with the patient. Especially when the patient is smiling and saying 'yes, yes', I carefully think about what that 'yes' means. If you do not listen attentively and dig for more information or confirm the patient's words, or ask opinions with an appropriate introduction, the interaction can easily take a structure like 'Please do whatever you want, doctor'.
リピートもパラフレーズもしないと、意図を読み取り違えていることもしばしばあるので、特に日本人はわからないとニコニコ誤魔化す。今日最初にお話された、男性の方なんかは、あの方も耳が遠くて、おそらく言ってた言葉は聞こえてなかったと思うんです。でも、あの状況で、聞き返したりとかしたら、失礼かもなと思って、ああ、はい、はい、って形で頷いたと思うんです。向こうが言ったことは聞き違えがないかの確認ができるけど、こちらが言ったことは伝わってるかどうかは意識しないと、笑ってハイハイと言われるとね、何のハイかなと思うんです。意識して少し掘り下げたりとか聞き直したりとか、枕詞を入れた上で意見をお聞きするとかしないと「先生のいいようにしてください」とそういう風になりやすくなるのは構造上あると思います。

13 I deliberately use a paternalistic style occasionally. 'I won't prescribe it to you because it's not suitable for you', I do it like this. Like today's case, the patient who requested the sleeping tablets. I say, 'I understand your feelings, but I think this is best'. I don't reject them without reasons.
あえてパターナリスティックにする時があります。「あなたには向かないから出しません」とか、そういう風にすることもあります。今日の睡眠薬のくだりとかね。あなたの気持ちもわかるんだけど、でも私はこうがいいと思うって。突っぱねたりはしませんけど。

Interview – D4

Researcher: Did you have communication skills training when you were a medical student?
医学部時代にコミュニケーショントレーニングはありましたか。

1 I don't remember much about [that in] medical school. Sometimes we watched videos of consultations with patients in a separate room in the department of general practice. When I was in the fifth year of medical school, I remember once we were asked to do real consultations, with the teacher and classmates observing, and we had feedback afterwards. We probably had a lecture on delivering bad news for cancer patients in a large lecture room, and only the students who raised their hands had a go. That's my impression. I did practice for OSCE with my friends many times, and we were doing it really being not sure of what was appropriate and what wasn't.
大学ではあんまり記憶にはないです。時々、総合診療で患者さんとのやり取りのビデオを別室で見られるとか。医学部の5年生の時に実際に問診をやってみましょうって、それを上の先生や同級生たちがみていて、あとでフィードバックみたいなのが一回あったのは覚えています。多分、大教室でガンの告知をやってみましょうとか、手を挙げた子だけやってみるような、そのくらいの印象です。OSCEの練習も友達同士で何度も練習して、それが適切なことなのか不適切なことなのかわかんないねって言いながらやってた感じです。

R: Do you think the style in which you communicate [with patients] has changed since then?
コミュニケーションスタイルは変わってきていますか?

2 Personally, I don't think I am good at communicating with people, because I grew up in a family where we didn't have much of this

back-and-forth mediation. Everyone just said what they wanted to say, and no matter what you said you wouldn't necessarily get a response to it. So I didn't get much of a basis for any communication style. [When I was a student], I was amongst people who shared the same background, for example, going to medical school from a metropolitan prep school, so we were able to skip over things and guess at what the other meant. But when I went into a job, I was like a fish out of water. I wasn't able to talk to patients properly, to start.
個人的にはコミュニケーションって常に得意ではないと思っていて、というのも、うちの実家がキャッチボールがあんまり成立しない家だったんです。みんな好き放題勝手なことをいう、何を言っても返ってくるとは限らないみたいなところがある家だった。基本的にはコミュニケーションスタイルがあんまりうまくできなくて。都内の進学校から医学部っていう、背景が同じような人の中でいたから、いろんなことを飛ばして話しても推察してくれたりとか、そういうところにいたので、就職した時に訳が分からなくなったんです。患者さんともそもそもうまく喋れないっていうか。

3 I'd mistakenly feel we'd already reached an understanding, or, otherwise, I'd intended to give a clear explanation which would then end up making no sense. I realised I was really bad at it, so after I became a resident, I started reading books about communication, and some books written by practitioners. So, I was looking for coaching methods and such. I still by no means think I'm great at it.
私的にはもう分かったような気がしてしまったり、逆に私の中でわかりやすく説明したつもりが、全然分からないになったり。本当に苦手だなって、研修医になってからコミュニケーションの本とか、臨床医の人の本を読んだりとかして、コーチングのやり方とか、模索していたし、今も決して上手だとは思わないので。

4 When I was a resident, I believed in medical knowledge strongly. For example, 'our information is correct if it is medically proven'. Looking at it positively, I had a strong sense of justice, but looking at it negatively, it was immature. I was very worried because – obviously – I didn't do well when I talked over patients' heads, showing off my medical knowledge. Through the process of my practice, I realised that the knowledge was not something to show off, and later, I began to learn the principles of a family physician, as well as from my own life events. I came to realise that it is always good to have various perspectives.
研修医の時は、医学的に正しいことは正しいという、よく言えば正義感が強く、悪く言えば未熟というか、知識を振りかざすタイプの考え方でした。伝わらない言葉で医学を振りかざしてもうまくいくはずはなくよく悩んでいました。やっていく中で、そもそも医学は振りかざすものではないんだとか、家庭医療の原則だったり自分自身のライフイベントもあったり、段々と色々あるのもいいんだという感じで。

R: Were you aiming for family medicine from the beginning?
最初から家庭医療のイメージを目指して来られたんですか。

5 I always wanted to be a generalist, but my university was strong in specialist training. They have a department for general practice, and it specialises in diagnostic, and is slightly different from the family medicine we do today.
総合的に診たいっていうのはずっとあったんですけど、うちの大学は専門色が強かったんです。総合診療科もあったんですけど、診断に特化していて、ちょっと今の家庭医療みたいなものとは違ったのね。

6 I wanted to try a variety of things, but that was all I knew when I was a student, so I was deciding between either psychiatry or paediatrics. I worked at a local hospital for the first two years of my training, and also practiced in a regional area, and in actual practice, I was sent to a rural infirmary, which I found interesting. I then learnt about family medicine, and I thought it was very close to what I wanted to do. That's how I ended up on this path.
でも色々みてみたい気持ちはあって、でも学生の時はそれしか知らなかったので、じゃあ精神科か小児科かどっちかと。最初の２年間の研修を地元の病院でやって、へき地医療もやって、実習で田舎の診療所に行かされて、面白いなあと思いました。家庭医療っていうのがあるんだって知って、これは私がなんとなく思い描いていたこういうのやりたいっていうことと近いなと思ってこの道に入ってきた。

R: I found your non-verbal styles very impressive, such as gazing or nodding, when listening to your patients.
先生の話を聞くときの目線とか頷き方とかノンバーバルの面が印象的です。

7 I used to rely too heavily on the verbal side a long time ago. Even though I studied hard to improve my verbal communication skills, I wasn't able to do it well, even using straight repetition. No matter how many times I used those techniques, they didn't work. I started thinking that it makes no sense to repeat while I'm still thinking that I want to persuade my patient somehow.
昔は、言葉に頼りすぎていたんだと思います。言葉をテクニック的にいろんなことを勉強しても結局うまくできなくて、おうむ返しにしましょうとか。いくらおうむ返ししても、結局どこかで説得してやろうみたいな意識の中でのおうむ返しは、しても意味ないのかなと思うようになりました。

8 I got divorced, and that was really tough. It was so painful for me. Partially, that is why I've been studying grief care. I was in deep shock

anyway, but I had to interact with patients even in those circumstances. After getting through that experience, I think I myself changed as a person. I thought that there isn't such a thing as only one thing being correct, and there are some things we cannot do anything about. It's the same for illnesses too, so, I stopped wanting to defer my actions to technical knowledge.
あと大きかったのは、一回離婚したこと。それはそれは大変だったんですよ。グリーフケアを勉強しているのもそれがあると思うんですけど、すごくショックを受けて、その状況の中でも患者さんとのやり取りはしなくてはいけなくて。そこを通り抜けた後に自分自身のありようみたいなものが変わったんだと思うんです。これだけが正しいとかそういうんじゃないんだなって、どうしようもないことってあるんだなって。それって病気も一緒だしって、そこでテクニックに頼ってどうこうとか、そういうことをしようと思わなくなったというか。

9 I found that it was important to think about what the patient is thinking in the background. I stopped thinking about little tricks for how to talk, and it turned out alright, as I felt able to do those little tricks in the end. Now I can express from my heart, 'I don't think so, but I see that you do think like that'. I have a feeling of respect for others who are different from me, like 'I cannot completely understand it, but it's been hard for you, right?' This is why I went back to graduate school to study again.
背景にどう思っているかというのが大事だと思うようになって、その小手先のことを考えなくなったら結果的に小手先の事もできるようになったという感じです。「私はそうは思わないけどあなたはそう思うんだね」というのが自然に言えるようになった。自分と違うものに対する敬意のようなものができたんじゃないかなと。「私には完全には理解できないけどあなたも大変なんですね」という。そういうこともあってわざわざ大学院にまた行って勉強しようと思ったのだと思う。

10 There is no one correct communication style. It's not my strong suit but would I do my best, in my own way. Maybe because of that, I felt I wanted to go back to university to study again. I think that the biggest change was within myself. Thinking about what I would be asked in this interview, I thought that I couldn't explain anything about my clinical communication if I leave out this event.
正解なコミュニケーションなんかないし、得意ではないけど自分なりにやって行こうって。そういうこともあって、わざわざ大学にまた行って勉強しようって思ったんだと思う。中身の自分が変わったというのが一番大きいと思う。インタビューで何を聞かれるのかなって考えて、コミュニケーションに関してこのことは、外してしまうと説明できないなと思って。

R: I often hear about doctors' burnout. I guess there are some cases of difficult patients.

医師のバーンアウトの話もよく聞きます。患者さんによって接するのが難しいケースありますよね。

11 That's right. Sometimes, I [my words] influenced the patient more than I thought, or I'm influenced. Some patients can be very aggressive when talking about their difficult situations, which makes you feel their pain. Now I'm able to recognise that it's their pain. I understand now that relationships do change over time. Even if I'm not always great at communication, I still try, looking to the long term.
そうなんです。自分 [の言葉] が思う以上に力を持って響いてしまったり、自分が影響されたり、辛い状態を攻撃するような形で言う患者さんもいるし、こっちが辛いなってなるけど。今は、ああ辛いんだなって、思えるようになって。関係って時間で変わっていくんだなって分かってきて、常に上手なコミュニケーションは出来なくても、長い軸ではなんとかやれるっていう感じになったかなって。

R: I was wondering who has the right to speak freely at your clinic…
先生のクリニックで発言権を持っている人というのは…

12 The practice head is in a strong position structurally, but it's a bit vague in terms of who everyone follows. There is a nurse who is kind and patient, and I feel that everyone trusts her. Also, the assistants are not medical workers, but from the general public, so they have common sense. I think that the long-serving assistants have people's trust (in the clinic).
現実的には事務長が構造的に強いんですけど、みんなが従ってついていってるかっていうと微妙で、看護師の中でソフトで粘り強い人がいて、その人のことはみんな信頼してるなっていう気がする。あとアシスタントたちは医療者ではなくて一般社会から来ているので常識的なんです。長くいてくれるアシスタントさんは信頼されているなと感じます。

13 Our practice is all on one floor, which is a leap I took because I wanted to create a flat structure [relationship-wise]. When I first joined this clinic, the doctor gave instructions to other staff, and the staff would help them, but then they'd keep saying they were doing it wrong. I think that we now all help each other. For example, an assistant can give the doctor a warning. It's a good thing. We can talk about non-work things, offer each other snacks, ask for pointers, that kind of thing. We can now talk more casually.
うちはワンフロアなので、あえてなんですけど、なるべくフラット [な関係性] にしたいねって希望して。私が最初ここに来た時は医者が指示を出して、他がサポートしていたけど、いやそうじゃないからって言い続けて。今はサポートし合えていると思います。アシスタントが医師に釘をさしてくれたりね。でもそれはいいことだと思ってます。お菓子食べますとか、関係ないことも話せたり。ちょっとこれ教えてとか。気軽に話せるので。

Interview – D7

Researcher: Did you want to become a family physician from the beginning?
最初から家庭医になりたいと希望されていたのですか。

1 Yes. My original motivation was to go in that direction, primary care and such. But it was vague. My specialism is in psychiatry. My university organises its medical departments according to organ groups, so if you do that, then there's no department of family medicine or general practice in the university. I thought it best to have some specialism, so, out of what was there at university, I thought ER was close, and went for that. There, I thought that any organ-based specialism seemed interesting, but I was also curious about the human ego, free will – nerve functions, on that sort of level.
そうです。元々のモチベーションはそっちの方向ですね、プライマリケアとか。漠然と思っていました。専門は精神科です。大学は臓器別の医局で団体がそれぞれあって、そういうのを見てると、家庭医療とか総合診療などは大学にはないんですね。何か専門性をもつ方がいいのではないかと思い、大学の中ではERですね、そこが近いかなと思って出入りしてたら、臓器別の専門の中ではどれも面白いと思ったけれど、自我とか、自由意志とか、そういうレベルの神経機能が面白いかなと興味を持って。

R: Do you think that the way that you communicate with patients changed during the interaction with patients since you started working here?
こちらで勤務を始めてから、患者さんとのやり取りの中でコミュニケーションが変わってきたと思いますか。

2 I think it's changed. I'm sure that there are differences in my skills, although I cannot say what's different. However, my skills are improving. In home visits, I change my style and approach depending on the particulars of each situation. Changing styles is usual for me, I suppose.
変わったと思います。スキルの部分は確実に違いはあるでしょうし、何が違うかというとわからないですが。ただスキルの方は好転しています。訪問診療はTPOでこっちの雰囲気を変えたりはします。自分のスタイルを変えること自体は元々ですかね。

3 For example, when I was in training in psychiatry, there were patients who were very excitable, severe hallucinations and such, who would come into the emergency psychiatry [ward] at night. They'd be in a

good mood, but they would've had a violent outburst and been caught by the police. I'd listen to them and asked why they were here, then they'd say, they felt so good at the train station, so they took off their clothes and made some noise. Listening to that makes you think that mania must feel really great, right? So I'd ask them if they felt great. And they'd say yes, they felt great.
例えば、精神科の研修を受けている時は、夜に精神科救急で幻覚妄想がひどいとか興奮の強い人が来る。機嫌はいいんだけど大暴れして警察に捕まって来るんです。話を聞いてると、今日はどうして来たんですかと聞くと、駅で心地よくなって裸になって大騒ぎしたっていうんですけど、話を聞くと、躁状態だと気分がいいんだろうなって思うんですよね。気分最高ですかって聞くんです。すると最高っていうんです。

4 Then, after that, I wouldn't go too far, but I would carry on the conversation, to elicit some information. Another style would be to make no moves at all. At the very least, some engagement is the first thing. Even if it's just a one-off after you've established a relationship. So when this shifts to a home environment, I adapt myself to the atmosphere there.
そうなったら、こっちも行きすぎることはないけれど、ある程度やり取りの連鎖をして、情報を引き出していくってことをしますね。こっちが全く動かないっていうスタイルでもいいんですけどね。少なくとも先ずはエンゲージメントですかね。関係作りから、一回きりであってもですね。ていう意味で、それが在宅の環境に移ったら、その雰囲気に合わせてやります。

5 Even I'm not really sure about what sort of communication styles belong to family medicine specifically. I don't know how communication differs between organ-specific practice and family [general] practice. There may be some difference. But this [adaptation] is something that definitely happens in home [family] practice.
何が家庭医的なコミュニケーションなのかは、自分の中でもちょっとわからないですね。臓器別の医療のコミュニケーションと家庭医のコミュニケーションとどう違うかがわからないです。あるのかもしれませんけど。実際、家庭において医療をする際には、確実にそうなりますね。

6 In an outpatient booth [in hospital], if a patient comes with family members, what the family says is very important. In terms of focusing on the family's story, my communication style is not that different. When visiting a patient's home, the place, as well as the people there, offers advantages. But, in terms of non-verbal communication, there are differences between hospitals and homes, so I utilise any information I can.
外来のブースに座っていて、家族が一緒に来る場合は家族の話が結構重要です。コミュニケーションスタイルはそれほど違わないです、家族へのフォーカスという意味では。家に行けば、人だけではなく、場の利点もあります。非言語的な意味でのコミュニケーションは病院と家では違うので利用できるものはします。

R: You are a specialist in consultations. I've heard a rumour that you're great at communication.
コンサルテーションにかけてはスペシャリストですよね。先生のコミュニケーションは良いよって噂を聞いています。

7 That may be true, in a sense. You could call me a specialist in actual clinical practice. Communication skills training is not included in Japanese medical education. Basically, the so-called 'OSCE generation' uses this one phrase 'That must have been hard'. I do not use this phrase often. It feels sympathetic. But [in medical school], everyone in my class was confused [when doing role-plays], because we all had to say that line and felt it may be rude instead. It does not sound caring. Empathy is more like identifying 'You think that …', right? Given that, what made us confused at that time was the sense that that ['That must have been hard'] was not the phrase to use.
ある意味ではそうかもしれないですね。実践の中でのスペシャリストと言っていいのかもしれないですね。コミュニケーションの教育というのは日本の医学教育にはないですから。基本的に、いわゆるOSCE世代は「それは大変ですね」ですから。僕はあまり使わない表現です。感覚としてはシンパシーです。それなのにその台詞を皆言うので、皆で混乱していたのです。むしろ失礼じゃないかと。他人事な感じがする。思ってないでしょって。エンパシーは「あなたはそう思っているんですね」になるんですよね。だとすると、学生の時に皆で違和感を感じていたのは、表現が違うってことですね。

Interview – D8

Researcher: It's been over 10 years since you graduated from medical school. Do you feel that the style in which you communicate [with patients] has changed since then?
卒後10年以上経ちますが、先生ご自身のコミュニケーションスタイルが変わってきたなという実感はありますか。

1 There's no huge change, but it has changed little by little as the years have passed. In hospital, I tended to follow treatment models, which occupied my mind and the contents of what I said. Patients expected it too to some extent. With home visits, my communication style leans more towards looking at the patient's lifestyle. In terms of finding the best way to discuss things, I try to improve [my skills] by looking to more experienced doctors or reflecting on things that I didn't handle too well. Compared to how I was when I'd just graduated, I think things go more smoothly now.

大きく変わったというのはないですけど、年次を重ねるにつれて少しずつ変わってきました。病院にいる時は医療モデルになりがちなんです。自分のマインドも喋る内容も。患者さんもそれを期待している部分もあります。在宅医療はより生活モデルに近いコミュニケーションの仕方になるかなと思います。どういう話し方がいいのかってのは、先輩の姿を見たりとか、実際に自分がうまくいかなかったことを振り返って改善したりっていうのはあります。卒業したての時に比べればスムーズにいくことは増えたと思います。

2 I wasn't fully aware of it, but I think various lectures I've attended have changed what I pay attention to. If I'd kept a record properly, I'd probably be able see the change. But I am not sure if I can call that a proper education in communication. We only did it once or twice. We also had simulated patients come in. But the core of it was not with simulated patients but amongst us students, alternating roles.
あまり自覚的ではないですけど、レクチャーを受けて意識するポイントが変わったり、おそらくちゃんと記録を取れば変わってきているんじゃないかなと思います。ただそれをコミュニケーションの授業と言っていいのかどうかです。本当に1回か2回、授業としてはやっただけだと思います。模擬患者さんが来たこともありました。ただ基本は模擬患者さんじゃなくて、学生同士で役割分担して。

R: Did you give feedback to each other?
フィードバックをしたり?

3 Yes, we did, but it was [only] simple. The palliative care training I received was more organised, and we had more solid feedback during that. If you're learning after you've graduated, you do tend to think that everyone is already doing [what's being taught], so you don't end up learning much. When I was a medical student, each one of the techniques was something new and revelatory for me.
そうですね。簡単なものでしたね。緩和ケア講習会の方が、そこはしっかりしていて、もう少しフィードバックがちゃんとありましたね。卒業してから習っても、もうみんな当然にやってるっていう思いもあるので、あんまり勉強にならない部分もあります。医学生の時はやっぱり、一つ一つの技法が新鮮でしたね、ああなるほどって。

R: Did you have any communication training when you were a medical student?
医学部時代にコミュニケーショントレーニングはありましたか。

4 I remember that we did medical interview practice in OSCE. There was a role-play, and I studied different cases that were likely to be included in the exam, reading textbooks. I'm not sure whether it was

OSCE or after graduation, but I remember I focused on practice for delivering bad news. Maybe it was in palliative care training.
記憶にあるのはOSCEですね。面談法、面接法を練習します。その中ではロールプレイもありましたし、こういうのが試験にでるからってケースで練習したり、教科書を読んで勉強したりしましたね。医学部生の時なのか卒業してからなのかちょっと記憶が曖昧ですけれど、悪い知らせを伝え方というのはとくに力を入れてやっていたと思います。もしかしたら緩和ケア講習会だったかもしれないですけどね。

5 What I remember now is that OSCE was just introduced when I was a medical student. [School] suddenly decided to do simulations, but even students who are confident in their communication skills don't do well in the simulations if they haven't learnt anything [about how to talk to patients], you know. This is what I learnt about the experience. We were eventually able to do it because we learnt to initiate a session with an open question, for example. But, if you haven't learnt it, you may likely start with a closed question for example.
医学部生の時に、OSCEの導入だと思うのですが、シミュレーションを急にやることになって、何にも習ってない状態だとコミュニケーションある程度自信がある人でもうまくいかないんです。それは非常に勉強になりました。まずオープンクエスチョンからとか、そういうのは習ったからこそできることだと思います。習わないと、いきなりクローズドクエスチョンで始まったりしがちだと思います。

R: Do you remember what textbooks you used in those days?
その当時どんな教科書を使っていたか記憶にありますか。

6 I think it went as far as the very few passages on medical interviews included in some chapters in those general OSCE prep books. I think we also had handouts from our teachers. In the general national exams, too, you do have to choose between techniques, closed questioning or active listening, for instance. They're easy questions, but since you do get asked those things, I did do some study for it from past papers and such.
よくあるOSCEの対策本とか、ごく一部の章に医療面接があるっていうくらいだったと思います。先生のハンドアウトもあったと思います。一般的な国家試験の対策の中でも、選択肢とかを出して、これはどの技法を使っているかとか、クローズドクエスチョンとか傾聴とか、簡単な問題ですけど、そういうのは聞かれるので、過去問で勉強したりもありますね。

R: I have the impression that education in Japan focuses on non-verbal behaviours, such as listening styles and postures. What do you think about this in practice?

日本では、傾聴のスタイルや姿勢など、言語化しない部分に教育がフォーカスしてる印象があるんですが、実際に先生はどう思いますか。

7 My impression is that the most common complaints from patients are: 'the doctor doesn't look at me when talking' or 'he only looked at the computer'. It's true that eye contact is important, but in reality, there are so many hospitals where doctors are busy reading electronic medical records. The national exam is conducted in written form rather than in actual practice, so even in the OSCE exam it has to be a question asking which technique is used for a given statement, rather than anything about whether there's eye contact or not.
私の印象としては患者さんからのクレームでよくあるのは「医者が目を見て話してくれない」とか「パソコンばかり見ている」とか。アイコンタクトが大切っていうのはそれはそうなんですけど、現実的には電子カルテをみるのに忙しい病院が多いんじゃないかと思います。国家試験も実技じゃなくて筆記なので、OSCEもどうしても問題文で訊くとなると、アイコンタクトの有無とかじゃなくて、この発言はなんの技法を使っているか答えなさいみたいな、そういう聞き方になっちゃうんですね。

8 I know that eye contact is really important, but I don't think I really pay attention to it. I think age has an influence too. Young doctors these days take the OSCE, but others who didn't do that have cultivated in their own ways, so it's very diverse. While some experienced doctors are very good, some do not care at all.
現実的にはアイコンタクトが大切なのはわかってるけど、すごく意識してやってるかっていうとそうでもないと思いますね。あと世代が影響すると思います。今の若い人たちはOSCEを受けてきてますけど、そうじゃない人は独自の方法なので、非常にバラバラというか、すごく上手なベテランの先生もいれば全然気にしてない先生もいると思います。

9 My university hospital used to be very small back when I was a student, although it has improved now. The meeting room for family members was always full and you couldn't use it. You had to separate off a corner of the nurse station with a curtain and have talks about finding cancer and such. It wasn't a calm atmosphere at all. But there just wasn't any other place to talk. I was jealous of other university hospitals that had many rooms.
私の大学のことで言えば、今はよくなりましたけど、僕が学生の時は病院すごく狭かったんですね。家族との面談室っていつも埋まってて使えなかったんですよ。ナースステーションの一角をカーテンで区切って、がんが見つかりましたみたいな話をするんですけど、全然落ち着かないですよね。でも場所がないのでしょうがないという感じでした。他の大学病院はたくさん部屋があっていいなって思いました。

10 My specialism was diabetes the whole time I was in the hospital, and now I do home visits looking at general internal medicine. The

patient's background is important, so I listened to it to a degree, but I had to see so many outpatients and only had three minutes for each patient. It was not enough time to touch the patient or listen to their heart, and I just looked at the data and wrote the record. Now, I visit four or five patients in the mornings, but when I had to see 30 patients in the hospital in the mornings, I couldn't listen to them, even though I wanted to. I had to write medical records as well. If there's a patient you want to listen to for longer, you really have to choose and decide 'just this one patient today', or you end up keeping patients waiting forever. If there's someone you just have to speak with, you can see them last, I suppose.
病院にいるときはずっと糖尿病を専門にやってきて、今も内科全般として在宅を見ているという形ですね。実際に社会背景も大切なので聞くことは聞くんですが、とにかく患者さんが多いので、外来は3分間くらいです。体にも触れないです。胸の音を聞く余裕もないですし、データだけ見て、カルテを書いて。在宅だったら午前中は4人か5人を診ますが、糖尿病の外来で30人みるってなると、聞きたくでも聞けないですからね。カルテも書かないといけないですから。もし長く話を聞きたい人がいるなら「今日はこの一人」みたいに決めるしかないですね。もしくは患者さんを延々と待たせるか。どうしても話したい人は最後にみるとかですかね。

11 At first, I did not like the situation, but through handling the workload from necessity, I learnt how I could make the patients feel satisfied even in a short time. Until then, I often focused on giving the information I wanted to tell, but I decided to reduce the ratio of talking as much as possible [and listened more]. This turned out well. Even though I really wanted to say something, I didn't say it if the patient was not ready to listen to me, and I spent more time listening instead. Otherwise, the patient would have no chance to speak during the three minutes.
最初はそういう短いのが苦手で嫌だったんですけど、必要に迫られてやってるうちに、短い時間でもどうやって満足してもらえるのか意識するようになりました。それまではこっちが話したいことを伝えるっていうことが多かったんですけれど、それを極力減らしたらうまくいくようになりました。本当は言いたくても、相手が聞く準備ができていなかったら、言わないでむしろ聞く時間を増やす。そうじゃないと相手も3分間何も話せないで終わってしまうので。

9.5 The Full Version of the Transcripts of Two Medical Consultations

Case 4

[00:00:00]

1 D Thank you in advance.
よろしくお願いします.

2 R Thank you in advance.
よろしくお願いします.
(2.0)

3 D The other day, you had blood in your urine again, didn't you?
((Potentially non-PCC: Starting with a closed question, D asks a lot of closed questions from Line 3 to Line 76.))
この間(.)血尿がまた出てしまったんですよね↑

4 P For two days.
二日間.

5 D Two days?
二日間↑

6 P After I took (the tablet),
飲んだら,

7 D Did it stop?
うん (.) 止まりました↑

8 P I took them for three or four days, but,
でも (.) 三日 (.) 四日くらい飲みましたけど,

9 D Right. Fosmicin, isn't it?
Didn't you have stomach-ache or anything like that?
うんうんうん (.) ホスミシンですね (3.0)
特にお腹痛いとかそういうのはなかったですか↑

10 P Not at all. It [just] suddenly…
全然なくって [ただ]パッと.

11 D [Right], right.
[うん.] うん.

12 P I went to the toilet, [and], um, [when I went,
トイレ行っ[て], あの (.) 下ろした[ら,

13 D [Right], right.
[うん], [はい.

14 P It suddenly,
パッとして,

15 D Right.
うん.

16 P After that, I thought [it can't be good that] there was blood
あとに, 血がついて[た, いけない]と思って,

17 D [Right, right.]
[うん,うん,]

18 P I [got] some tablets [and] took them for three days.
お薬[を]いただい[て], 三日飲みました.

19 D You [took] them for three days.
[はい.][ええ.]

三日飲みまし[た.]
20 P [Yes.]
[はい.]
21 D Before, I asked you to >please collect a sample,<
I think it was a plastic bottle, and
what came out was pretty much pure red,
前は (.) ペットボトルだったかしら,
>とっておいていただいてね,<
結構真っ赤なのが出てましたけど,
22 P Yes.
はい.
23 D Was this time less than last time?
この間ほど量は多くなかった↑
24 P <Yes.>
<そうなんです>.
25 D There wasn't that much?
そんなに多くはなかった↑
26 P It only happened just once
一回だけ (.) でただけで,
27 D Just once.
一回だけ,
28 P There was [nothing] after that.
あとは[なんでも]なくて,
29 D [Right.] Previously, you had it every three months, but
this time the period was a bit shorter, [it happened again]
right away,
[うんうん.]
(3.0) 今までね (.) 三ヶ月おきにそういうことがあったんですけど,
今回はちょっと (.) 短かった (.) すぐ[にまた,]
30 P [hh Yes, it was shorter.
[.hh 短かかったですね.
31 D >Has that happened before?<
>そういうことって前もありました↑<
(2.0)
32 P It hasn't.
ありません.
33 D It hasn't?
Right. So previously it was about three months.
なかったです↑
うんうん (.) 今までは三ヶ月くらいだったんですね.
34 P Exactly. [Well, bleeding hadn't happened before,
全くね (.) その出血するということは (.) なかった[んです,
35 D [It hadn't. I see.
[なかったんですね. うん.
(2.0)
36 P That [started] two or three years ago,
それが二, 三年前から (.) 出る[ようになって,]
37 D [I see.]
[そうですね.]

38 P After it started, it happened once every three [or six months,
そうしたら (.) 三ヶ月にいっぺんくら[い：半年くらい,

39 D [I see.]
Initially, it happened once every six months, but
the interval is getting a bit shorter?
[そうですね.] 最初は半年にいっぺんだったのが,
ちょっと間隔が短くなってきてます↑

40 P This time was shorter.
今度は短かった.

41 D So this time was shorter.
It was at the beginning of February, right? Right,
[so, about a month.
今回はね, 短かったですね.
二月の頭でしたもんね？そうですよね, 一ヶ月くらい[ですね.

42 P [Yes.] (5.0)
I [was told] to drink water,
[そう.]
で (.) 水を飲むようにって[ご注意をいただいた,]

43 D [Right.] Yes, yes.
[うんうん.] はいはい.

44 P so, I drank more and more water. (2.0)
It disappeared about two days later.
だからどんどん水を飲んでました.
二日くらいで (.) 何でもなくなって.

45 D Right. Have you been urinating more frequently than before, or
do you have pain when you urinate? Any symptoms like that?
((multiple questions))
うん. おしっこが今までよりも (.) 頻繁に出るとか,
おしっこする時に痛いとか (.) そういうのはなかったですか↑

46 P It['s] not painful, but it is frequent.
痛くはないで[す.] でも頻繁ですね.

47 D [I see.] It's frequent?
[うん.] 頻繁↑

48 P Well, with a lot of water,
あの (.) どんどん水を,

49 D Since you drink a lot of water. Right, right.
いっぱい飲むからね, うんうん.

50 P But I'm not sure whether there was,
が (.) あったかどうか,

51 D Well, it's the same as normal, which [was] frequent
to begin with, and it hasn't changed, has it?
((It has taken many closed questions to clarify the patient's history – this could be potentially non-PCC; However, this could also show that the doctor assists well the patient in recollecting the event))
ま (.) いつもとは変わらない (.) もともと頻繁に (.) [あって,]
変わらないということですね↑

52 P Yes. [(hh)]
はい.

53 D How about feeling residual urine?
Have you had anything like that?
残尿感とか (.) そういうのもなかったです↑
54 P I haven't felt like there was residual urine.
I've [never] felt that before.
残尿感はないんです.
今まで[も一度も], それはないんです.
55 D [You haven't.] Okay, how about your physical condition
such as your appetite, have there been any changes?
[なかった.] じゃ体調とかそういったところ (.) 食欲とか (.) そう
いうのも,
全然お変わりないですか↑
56 P Yes (hh), I'm eating a lot.
はい(hh). よく食べてる.
57 D You're eating a lot.
よく食べてる.
(2.0)
58 D Last time, you said your back pain was getting much better.
How is it feeling now?
この間ね (.) 腰の痛みがだいぶいいですよっておっしゃってた[
けど,]
今はどうかしら↑
59 P [Ah, yes.] It hurts again,
[あ, はい.]
また痛くて,
60 D Right.
うん.
61 P It was very painful yesterday and the day before,
for two days straight.
昨日 (.) おとといか (.) 二日続けて (.) も : : う痛くて痛くて,
62 D Right.
うん.
63 P I said I was going to make hamburgers and [went] to
the kitchen, but, I couldn't (hh) do it [and]
ate something else.
あ, ハンバーグを作るって言って台所へ[行って,]
もう (hh) 作れなく[て,] 違うもの食べて.
64 D [Right,] [right.]
[うん.] [うん.]
65 P Last night, (9.0) I wanted to eat something,
夕べは, (9.0) 何食べようと思ったのかな,
66 D Right.
うんうん.
67 P but I just [went] to bed because it was so painful.
痛くて痛くて (.) 寝ちゃいまし[た.
68 D [Right.] Did you use a painkiller?
[うん.] 痛み止めは使いました↑
69 P Yes.
はい.

70 D Which one did you use? The tablets?
どっちを使ったかしら (.) 内服↑

71 P Just the tablets. It wasn't bad enough to need
a suppository yet.
飲むのだけ. まだ座薬を入れるほどのことはなかった.

72 D Did you take it two times?
How many tablets did you use throughout the day, one?
Two?
((multiple questions))
二回くらい↑ 一日に一錠, 二錠 (.) どれくらい使いました↑

73 P Oh, I [took] it two times.
あ, 二回 (.) 飲み[ました.]

74 D [You took it two times?
[二回飲みました↑

75 P Yes.
はい.

76 D Did you take it today?
今日は飲みました↑

77 P I [haven't] taken it today (hh),
because it's not hurting [yet].
今日(hh)は飲んでま[せん (.) まだ]痛くないんで.

78 D [You haven't taken it today.] Right, right.
(2.0)
[今日は飲んでない.] うんうん.

79 P Should I take it only when it hurts, or
should I be taking it consistently?
痛いときだけ：しょっちゅう飲んでた方がいいんですか↑

80 D >No, I suggest you take it only when it hurts.<
>いや痛いときだけの方がいいと思います.<

81 P Oh, my stomach starts to hurt right after I take it,
なんかね (.) すぐ胃が痛くなったり,

82 D I see.
そうですね.

83 P [so because] of that, um, I only take it when it hurts,
ていうことに[なるんで,] あの (.) 痛いときだけ飲んで,

84 D [Right, right.] I see. It's best to take it just when it hurts,
because the medication itself has some side effects.
[うんうん.]
そうですね (.) 痛いときだけの方がいいですね,
副作用がそれなりにあるのでね.

85 P Yes.
はい.

86 D It's not something you use consistently for a long period.
長いことず：っと (.) 使うものではないのでね.

87 D Okay, we talked about rehabilitation last time.
Did you talk to your care manager about wanting to try it?
はい. この間 (.) リハビリの↑ (.) お話：をしたら,
リハビリちょっとやってみようかなってお話が,
ケアマネさんにありました↑

88	P	Yes. はい.
89	D	It seems you're feeling a bit more motivated about it. ((acknowledging her motivation about walking)) ね, 少し (.) やる気になったのかしら.
90	P	I think I want to try walking. 歩いてみようかと.
91	D	Oh, really? Right, right. あ, 本当ですか. うんうん.
92	P	[Someone] who walked [with me] before was here, に (.) [一緒に]歩いてくれた[方が]いらっしゃったんで =
93	D	[Right.] [Yes, yes.] [ええ.] [はい, はい.]
94	P	I talked to my care manager about it [and, =ケアマネージャーの[方に] (.) お話し[て,=
95	D	[Right.] [Yes. [ええ.] [うん.
96	P	Then, =それで, また少し.
97	D	I see. そうですか.
98	P	But, it's not ideal when it's so cold. でもあん : まり寒い時はね : :
99	D	Yes, that's right. ((understanding the difficulty in walking in the winter)) うん, そうですね.
100	P	Once it gets warmer outside. Um, we talked about that, so, ちょっとあったかくなったらね. あの (.) 話しておきましたので,
101	D	Right, then, around when the cherry blossoms bloom, ((visualising walking in the nice weather from the patient's perspective)) あ,そうですか (.) じゃ (.) 桜が咲いたらとか,
102	P	hhh ((laugh))
103	D	Right? Around when the weather gets nicer. ね, いいお天気になってきたら (.) とかね.
104	P	Yes. そうですね.
105	D	Once the weather gets nice enough that you want to take a stroll, it would be great if you could start around then. Yes. ((showing understanding; combination of positive and negative face. The last utterance is attending negative face: giving space to the patient.)) お散歩したくなってきたらね. 始められるといいですね (.) うんうん.
106	D	Well, I will start the physical examination then. ((preparation)) じゃ (.) ちょっと診察をさせていただきますね.

[00:06:29]
(6.0)
107 D Let's take off your shirt.
じゃ一枚脱ぎましょうかね.
108 P I'm sorry I'm in my pyjamas.
I should change my clothes when you come to visit, but,
パジャマのまんまでごめんなさい.
来ていた-だ-くんだから (.) 着替えないといけないんだけど,
109 D It's fine (hh). It's your home here. Wear whatever you like.
いえいえ (hh) おうちだから (.) 好きな格好でね.
(58.0)
((measuring blood pressure))
110 D 165, 60. [That's a little,
165の60です. [ちょっと,
111 P [Oh, it's high.
[あ, 高い.
112 D Yes, it is.
Do you measure your blood pressure at home? What is it usually?
ね. おうちで測ってますか?どれくらいかしら↑
113 P Just before- just before I measured it [and] it was 126.
さっきは- さっきはかっ[てね,] 126.
114 D [Right.] Oh, 126. Ah, I see.
[うん.] おお : 126. ああ, そうですか.
115 P Over 59.
下が59.
116 D Oh, I see. It's <u>great</u> that you remember it (hh).
((praise))
おお : そうですか. よく覚えてらっしゃいますね, <u>さすがです</u> (hh).
117 P It's because I've just measured it.
測ったばっかりだから.
118 D If those are your numbers at home, then you're just fine.
[This is…]
おうちでそれくらいの血圧であれば (.) ちょうどいいですので : ,
[こういうの,]
119 P [I see.] Doctor, as high as 160…
((P sounds concerned)
[そうですか.] 先生, 160なんて,
120 D This is called <“white coat hypertension”>. White coat.
That's the name for [when] you have high blood pressure
only when it's measured by a doctor, but it just means
you're nervous.
こういうのは<白衣高血圧>っていうんですよね. 白衣.
お医者さんが図ると高い[っていう,]
名前がついてるんですけど, 緊張してるの.
121 P You make me nervous.
((P shows humour)) [(hhh)]
£先生がいけない£.
122 D £ Yes, I make you nervous £.
£そう私がいけない£.

123 P hhhh
124 D You rushed here, right?
(hh) 急いで来たじゃない.
125 P Because you're beautiful.
((joke))
先生が美人だから.
126 D No, no, no. Thank you. hh.
いやいやいや (.) £ありがとうございます£ hh
127 P hhhh
128 D You rushed just now, because you were told to
'come right away'. You rushed, so you were out of breath, yes.
I think that also influenced your blood pressure and
made it higher.
急いで来たでしょ. 今ほら来なさいって言われて,
急いで来たでしょ今. それで (.) はあはあってなっちゃったし, うん.
そういう影響もあってね, 高いんだと思いますよ.
129 P Yes. But, don't you think the doctor is very beautiful?
((talks to the researcher))
ね, でも先生ね, すっごい美人だと思いません↑
130 R I think so.
思いますよ.
131 D No, no. Are you ready? Nothing will come out of it,
but, hhh ((laugh))
(22.0) ((pulse oximeter))
£いや, 大丈夫ですか£. hhh 何も出ませんけど hhh
132 D 96%. It's fine.
There's no problem if it's above 95. It's okay.
96%ね. 大丈夫です.
95以上あれば問題ないのでね. オッケーです.
133 P Your mole, here, looks charming.
ね, 先生の (.) £ここのほくろ, チャーミング£.
134 D Oh, really? This one under the eye.
あ (.) 本当↑ 涙ぼくろね.
135 P hhh ((laugh))
136 D hhh ((laugh))
137 D I'm going to listen to your heart sounds.
お胸の音聞きますよ：.
138 P Okay.
はい.
(21.0)
139 D And now to your back.
はいじゃあお背中ですね.
(4.0)
140 D Okay, breathe in and out [...] Nicely done.
はい, 息を吸って：吐いて [...] いいですよ.
141 D Do you feel pain here? Or here?
How about your stomach?
こういうところは痛くないですか↑ こういうとこも痛くない↑
お腹も痛くはないです↑

142 P My stomach doesn't hurt.
お腹は痛くない.
143 D It doesn't hurt.
痛くない.
144 P Yes.
はい.
145 D How about your bowel movement?
お通じはどうですか↑
146 P Today- today I had a big one.
今日は- 今日はすごくありました.
147 D Today you did. Really.
Well, things seem to be moving well then.
The movements inside. Um.
今日はありました. 本当. じゃ動きもいいですね : .
中の動きもね : Um.
(4.0)
148 D Have you had a cold, or anything like that?
なんか風邪ひいてたとか (.) そういうこともなかったです ↑
149 P I don't think so. (4.0) But I sneeze a lot and
ないと思うんです. (4.0) でも (.) すごくくしゃみしたり=
150 D Right, right.
うんうん.
151 P then my eyes water, and
=それから涙がでたり=
152 D Right, right.
うんうん.
153 P my eyes itch, but,
=目が痒かったりするんですけど,
154 D That sounds like hay fever.
花粉症みたいですね (.) それね.
155 P I don't think I've caught a cold.
風邪は引いてないと思うんですけど.
156 D In terms of symptoms, it's similar to hay fever.
The itchy eyes and sneezing,
Have you had those symptoms before?
ちょっと症状としては花粉症に似てますけど.
目の痒みとね, くしゃみとかね,
今まではそういうのはなかったです↑
157 P I've never really noticed hay fever before.
あんまり花粉症っていうの (.) 意識したことないんですけど,
158 D You haven't. I see. Well, your heart sounds are good,
and your lung sounds are good as well.
なかった. そうですか. まあお胸の音も綺麗だし,
肺の音も綺麗ですし,
159 P Oh, good. I'm [relieved.
あ (.) そうですか. 安心[しました.
160 D [You're just fine.
[特に問題はないですね.
161 P I'm relieved.

安心しました.
162 D Right.
(4.0)
はい.
[00:12:25]
163 D Then, you should still have four days of antibiotics left,
right? Um, you should have four days left of the Fosmicin,
the medicine for your cystitis.
じゃ抗生剤はまだ (.) 4日分はあるのかしらね.
あの (.) ホスミシン, ホスミシンていう, 膀胱炎の時のお薬は,
まだ4日分[は,
164 P [Yes, I have it.
[あります.
165 D You have it. Good, good.
ありますかね. うんうん.
166 D Your previous doctor. Did he tell you that
once you start taking it, you need to take it
for seven consecutive days and finish it? Were you told that?
これ前の先生にはね (.) 先生には,
1回飲み始めたら7日間で飲みきるようにって言われませんでした↑
言われてない↑
167 P He [might have said that (hh). ((laugh))
おっしゃった (hh) かも [しれない.
168 D [Might have.
So, basically, [once your symptom stopped,
[しれない.
あの：本来は症状がおさまった[ら,
169 P [But, that doctor…
((cutting in))
[でもね, あの先生ね,
170 D Yes.
うん.
171 P he said I don't need tablets!
((making a sound as if the former told her off))
薬はいらんって言って,
172 D That's right. Drinking water is more important.
そうそうそう. お水飲むほうが大事.
173 P He said 'drink water'
水飲んでなさいって,
174 D That's right. That's one thing you can try, but next time,
you might find it's the same whether you take antibiotics
or not. If it's cystitis, you don't actually need to take tablets,
because, as the doctor said, drinking water should cure it.
((D continues to explain and educate P))
そうですね. ま (.) それでやってみてもいいかもしれないですけどね,
次回ね (.) 同じかもしれない. 抗生剤を飲もうが, 呑まなかろうが,
膀胱炎だったら, 本当はお薬はいらないので,

先生のおっしゃる通りでお水飲めば治るはずだから.
175 P ((silent))
(3.0)
176 D meaning, antibiotics, if you take them,
ていうのは, 抗生剤はね, あの飲めばね,
177 P Huh...
なんかね=
178 D Yes.
うん.
179 P After I took the tablets for three days,
my stomach felt heavy, and I didn't feel like
eating anything, [I just slept.]
((P's showing what happened to her after taking antibiotics,
which she has not shared before))
=あの3日間飲んでたら[ね, 胃が重苦しい感じがして,]
なんかなんにも食べたくないし, [で寝てたんですね.]
180 D [Right, right.]
[うんうん, うんうん.]
181 P So, I thought it was no good to keep taking them.
だからこれじゃあダメだろうと.
182 D Yes, I see. There are some side effects.
With medicine, if you stop taking it partway through,
well, have you heard of 'resistant bacteria'?
うんうん, そうですね. それなりに副作用もあるし,
お薬をね, こう中途半端に飲んでしまうと,
耐性菌って聞いたことあります↑
183 P I haven't.
知りません.
184 D They're bacteria that become stronger than the medicine,
あの：菌がね, 薬よりも強くなってしまったね,
185 P Ah- I see.
あ- はい.
186 D and in the future, the medicine might become ineffective, so
it's said that you shouldn't take antibiotics
if you're going to take them incorrectly.
将来ね, 効かなくなる可能性があるから,
抗生剤はむやみやたらにはのまないほうが,
いいって言われてるんですよね.
((reeducation))
187 P Right.
はい.
188 D This means that if you plan to take it, you should take
it properly for the whole week, and, if you don't plan
to take it fully, you should take none at all. Meaning,
either zero days or seven days is the way to do it, so,
((D has given so much information and general advice; these
also appear too prescriptive: potentially non-PCC))
そういう意味では, 飲むんだったら一週間しっかり飲んだ
ほうがいいし,

のまないんならもうのまないどっちかですね.
ゼロか7日間かっていう感じでね (.) やったほうがいいので,

189 P I was careless.
不注意でした.

190 D No, no. It's no problem, no problem at all.
I just think we should try it like that [next time].
((seeking mutual agreement))
いえいえ (.) いいんですいいんです.
そういう風に今度[から,] しようかなって思うんですけど,

191 P Yes.
[はい.]

192 D Then, shall we try just water next time?
If you don't have a stomach-ache or any symptoms like that,
just drink water even if you have blood in your urine,
そしたら次回は, お水だけでやってみます↑
特にお腹痛いとか症状なければ, 血尿出てもお水だけ飲んで=

193 P Yes.
はい.

194 D without taking antibiotics, shall we try that?
=抗生剤は呑まないで, やってみます↑

195 P I'll try that.
やってみます.

196 D Let's do it.
やってみましょうか.

197 P Yes.
はい.

198 D Right. But if you continue to have blood in your urine
even after that, we'll start taking antibiotics again. Okay.
うん (.) それでもやっぱり止まらないってことであれば,
飲み始めましょうかね, うん.

199 P Um. I'll call you,
あの (.) 電話,

200 D Right.
うん.

201 P on the phone.
させていただきます.

202 D Okay. Yes, that's fine.
そうですね, はい. わかりました.

203 P Thank you.
よろしくお願いします.

204 D Yes, you're welcome.
Then, today I won't give you a prescription.
Is that okay with you?
はい (.) よろしくお願いします.
じゃ今日はお薬は (.) 特に出しませんけど大丈夫ですかね.

205 P Do I still have that medicine to sleep? [My husband has it.]
あの眠る薬は,まだありますか↑ [主人が持ってるんで.]

206	D	[Yes. Right, right.] [うん. ええ, ええ.]
207	P	I don't know how much is gone or how many tablets are left though.] 私は, どんだけ減ってるんだか, あと何錠あるんだか知らないんですけど.
208	D	I see. Let me see, last time, Ebamiru, なるほど, ええとね, 前回エバミールね, ((D does not appear to ask about P's sleeping: e.g., how's your sleep?))
209	P	Yes. はい.
210	D	I prescribed it for four weeks, so, 4週間分出してるので,
211	P	Yes. はい.
212	D	that should be enough even if you take two every day. 二錠ずつ毎日飲んでも足りてるはずです.
213	P	Okay. はい.
214	D	I can prescribe it again next time, so, また次回処方の日なので,
215	P	Next time, 次回,
216	D	On the 19th 19日.
217	P	It will be okay until you come next time. 来ていただくまでは大丈夫.
218	D	Yes. 大丈夫.
219	P	Seems like it will be enough. ありそう.
220	D	Is there anything else you need? 大丈夫です↑
221	P	No. はい.
222	D	Then, I'll see you in two weeks. じゃあまた二週間後ね. [close the session]
223	D	Alright, I'll be back in two weeks. Give me a call if there's anything you need. はいじゃあ, 2週間後に伺いますので, 何かあればご連絡ください.
224	P	Thank you very much. ありがとうございます.

Case 17

[00:00:00]
1 N Then, let me measure your body temperature first.
はいじゃ：：先にちょっとお熱を測りますよ：.
2 P Okay.
はい.
((N checks vital signs))
(9.0)
3 D How are you doing? ((Indication of PCC: open question))
調子はどうですか↑
4 P Um, not much has changed…
う：：ん：あんまり変わらないんだよな：：.
5 D Um… How's your back?
((semi-open question allowing the patient to answer at some length about the pain))
Um：腰の塩梅はどうです↑
6 P Well, only for my back, it [doesn't hurt anymore.
あのね, そこだけはね, [痛くなくなった.
7 D [I see. Ah, that's good. I see.
((encouragement))
[ええ,
あ, £それは良かった£. そうですか.
8 P It seems like the medication made the,
what should I call it, the film-like thing go away.
なんていうかな,
膜- みたいなの[が,] 薬のせいでなくなったらしいんだよ.
9 D [Yes.] I see, I see.
[はい.] はいはい, ええ, ええ.
(5.0)
10 P After I talked to the nurse last time, she said it's all clean.
この間, 看護師と話した[後, 綺麗になりましたよって,
11 D [Yes.] Ah, I see. Right, right, right.
[ええ. あ：：そうですか, ええ, ええ, ええ.
(3.0)
12 D By the way, I haven't seen your <wife> recently.
Is she still the same as always?
((D's showing interest in P's world by including a topic about wife))
そういえば私最近, <奥様>お会いしてませんけど,
奥様の方も (.) 特別お変わりは,
13 P Yes, I don't think anything's changed.
ないと思います.
14 D I see. That's good. ((encouragement))
そうですか (.) 何よりでした.
(6.0)
15 N 98, 83.
16 D 98, 83. ((writing it down))
Have you been able to <eat> well?
<お食事は>しっかり食べれますか↑

17	P	Well, now, I've been asking for my rice to be cut down to about 70% of what it was. そう：ね：今ご飯を[ね,] 七分目くらいにしてもらってるんですよ.
18	D	[Right.] Ah, I see. [Can you finish that much? [ええ.] ああそうですか (.) 七分目だと全部きれいに食べれ[ます↑
19	P	I can usually finish the [side dishes. [おかずはね, だいたい (.) 食べられる.
20	D	You're finishing the side dishes. おかずは全部召し上がってる.
21	P	Yes. はい.
22	D	I see. It's only rice you've cut down to 70%. ああ. ご飯だけちょっと七分目に,
23	P	Yes, yes, yes. そうそうそう.
24	D	Aha. ((writing it down)) あ：　は：： (5.0)
25	N	>Okay, I'm going to measure your blood pressure. Let's take off just this one.< >じゃあね血圧を測るので (.) こっちだけ脱ごうかな.<
26	P	Okay. はい. (4.0)
27	N	It's a bit cold today, isn't it? 今日はちょっと寒いですもんね.
28	P	[Yes, a bit cold. ちょっと寒い[ね.
29	N	Yes. [ね：：. (9.0)
30	P	Doctor, at night, I still… ((initiation of a topic)) 先生やっぱり夜はね：：=
31	D	Yes. はい.
32	P	I can't sleep the whole time. =ずーっと寝られないんですよ.
33	D	You can't sleep. I see… 寝られない (.) うん：：.
34	P	I sleep for two hours, and like this… 2時間くらい眠ってこう,
35	D	Ah, you fall asleep and [wake up. あ：：寝て, 目が[覚めて,
36	P	[Yes, yes, yes. [そうそうそう.

37	D	Then fall asleep and wake up again. I see. また寝て,目が覚めて (.) ああ : : .
38	P	When I wake up, その覚めた時に : =
39	D	Yes はい.
40	P	Well, I feel like going to the toilet. =あの : : トイレ行きたくなっちゃうんですよね.
41	D	Ah, I see, I see. あ (.) なるほどなるほど.
42	P	I wake up to go to the toilet over and over. トイレで起きる, [それが] こう繰り返して,
43	D	[Right,] right. [うん.] うん.
44	P	They (nursing home) offer dinner early. あそこはね : 夕食は早んですよ.
45	D	I see. は : は : .
46	P	5 or 6 o'clock. 5時から6時[か.
47	D	Ah, that's early. I see. [あ : 早めですね, うん.
48	P	So, everything is done at around 6:30. だから6時半頃には (.) もうみんな終わっちゃってさ,
49	D	I see… うん : : .
50	P	Which means I just <zone out>. <ぼやーん>としてるわけよ.
51	D	hhhh
52	P	People who want to sleep do so at 7, 寝たい人は7時には,
53	D	Oh, that's pretty early. あ, 結構早くから,
54	P	Yes. うん.
55	D	What time do they <turn off the lights>? <消灯>みたいな時間は,
56	P	It's about 8. だいたい8時.
57	D	About 8. だいたい8時.
58	P	Yes. うん.
59	D	Well, that sounds early too (hh). Umm. Do you go to bed and sleep at 8? Already by around 8 in the evening, まあそれでも早いなって (hhh) 感じですかね. Umm : : 8時に床について (.) 横になって休むんですか↑ 夜8時くらいにはもう,

60 P Ah, at that place (the nursing home).
あ：：向こうでね.

61 D I see.
ええ.

62 P Nothing I can do about it.
しょうがないもん.
(4.0)

63 D Your blood pressure is around 100 or 110…
((checking his blood pressure. Writing and checking records))
血圧だいたい100, 110.
(17.0)

64 P In the morning,
朝がね,

65 D Yes.
はい.

66 P I wake up at around 5.
だいたい5時に起きるんですよ.

67 D Ah…
あ：：.

68 P It's early.
早いんだ.

69 D Right.
うん
(11.0)

70 P Breakfast is at 7.
朝食は：：7時かな.

71 D It starts at 7. Um.
7時から. Um：.

72 P Lunch starts at 11.
昼食が11時から.

73 D Right. (2.0) I see.
うんうん. (2.0) なるほど.
(3.0)

74 P There's not much time between them.
この間が早んだよね.

75 D I see. Um. Well, shall I listen to your heart sounds?
((listening to his heart sounds))
そうですね. Um：：ちょっと胸の音を聞きましょうか.

76 P Okay. (8.0) All of it, from top to bottom, that- that.
はい. (8.0)
全：：部, 上から下まで (.) あちらの- あれです.

77 D Okay, they do (wash clothes).
It's helpful that they wash your clothes and such.
Make them nice and neat.
あ, やっていただいて.
でも, お洋服とか助かりますね. きれいに (.) なって.

78 P Yes, yes.
そうそう.
(18.0)

79 D Let's listen to your <back>.
((listening to his lung sounds))
<背中>の音を聞きましょう.
(10.0)
80 D Okay, thank you.
はい (.) ありがとうございます.
81 P Yes.
はい.
82 D At night, is the toilet far away from the room where you sleep?
夜は, トイレは (.) その寝る部屋からは離れてるんですか↑
83 P No, I bring the portable one,
いやあの (.) ポータブルを持ってきて,
84 D Ah, you use that one at night,
あ, 夜はそちらを使って,
85 P By the bed.
ベッドの脇で.
86 D By the bed. Right.
脇で. うんうんうん.
[00:05:36]
87 D Right. I see. So, for example,
medicine that helps you sleep a little better at night,
そうでしたか. まあ例えばですけど,
夜その : : もう少し寝つきをよくする薬とかを,
88 P Yes.
はい.
89 D like when we tried it before when you were staying at home,
such medicines [make you] feel dizzy
if you wake up in the middle of the night.
使う方法もあるんですが,
前もその : : おうちに普段いらっしゃる時に,
ちょっと試したこともあるように, 寝つきをよくする薬は,
ちょっと夜中とかに逆に目が覚めると : ふらふら[しちゃったり]
とか=
90 P [Dizzy, right.]
[ふらふらね.]
91 D or make you fall more easily… so they're,
=転びやすかったり : : ちょっと,
92 P Um, well,
Um (.) あのね,
93 D There are risks like that as well, so
taking medicine is not necessarily a better choice. [Um…
((explains a risk))
そういう危ないとこもあって,
飲んだらいちがいにいいかっていうと,
必ずしもそうじゃないかもしれません. [Um : : .
94 P Yes, yes, yes.
[はいはいはい.
95 D Um. Among the prescription you have now,
one of them helps you sleep more deeply.

That one rarely has side effects such as feeling dizzy,
so it can be used safely even by older adults, [but,
Um : 今もお薬は一つ (.) あの,
他の薬と混ぜて, 寝つきを深くするお薬入れてるんですが,
そのお薬は, う : : んと : : いわゆるフラフラとかですね,
副作用はほとんどないので,
年配の方でも安心して使える薬なんです[けど,

96 P Ah, I see.
[あ (.) そうですか.

97 D If you were to use another tablet rather than this one
being sleepy means you feel drowsy, so if you feel like
going to the toilet in the middle of the night,
you might walk unsteadily, which is dangerous.
So you could say there are < two sides > to it. Yes…
((D has explained any possible risks and emphasises both positive and negative sides))
この薬じゃない他の薬を使うっていうと,
眠気がするってことはこう, うつらうつらするっていう意味なので,
ちょっと夜中にトイレに行こうと : : 思ったらきっと,
フラフラっとするとかですね,
そういう危険性と, <表裏の関係>って言いますか. うん : .

98 P Then, is the current one okay?
じゃあ今のやつだったら (.) 大丈夫↑

99 D This one is fine.
今のやつだったら大丈夫です.

100 P Ah. Then, could I get one more?
((P's request for extra tablets))
あ. じゃそれもう一つ増やしてもらおうか.

101 D It- it's >not a medicine that I can< give more of.
One- The amount of the medicine is fixed. Um…
増や- 増やすのはね (.) >できない薬なんですよ<. それは.
一つって- 量が決まってる薬なので. Um : .

102 P Look, it's not like I walk to the toilet, [so
it's right here, [so,
So, I don't think you need to worry about that, but…
((P seems positive about managing with being drowsy from an extra tablet))
トイレほら : 行く訳じゃないから,
ここにある[から, だからその点は安心だなと思うけど.

103 D [Yes. Yes.] I see…
[う : : ん (.) う : : ん.]
そうですね : : .

104 P I'll leave the decision to you.
先生のご判断に任せます.

105 D Hmm…
((checking his medical history; D's taking consideration rather than denying immediately, which takes 37 seconds))
う : : ん.
(37.0)

106 D I've taken another look at what medicines you're taking currently…
今の, 飲んでる薬とかをもう一度点検して見てみましたけど,

107 P Yes.
はい.

108 D Um… after considering the possibility of side effects, I wouldn't [recommend using any additional medicine.
う : : ん. その副作用の可能性を考えると,
そういう追加でお薬を使うのは, 私はやめた方がいいと思い[ます.

109 P [Right. I understand.
[はい.
わかりました.

110 D Right… well, I really understand how you feel.
I think they turn the lights off early (at the nursing home), but (hh), ((laugh))
う : : ん. まあ, お気持ちもよく分かりますし,
暗くなるのが早いなと思いますけど (hh),

111 P Yes.
はい.

112 D I bet it's not easy to sleep, even though they turn out the lights at 8. Um. But I think it's better to avoid it.
((D's emphasising "avoid it"))
£8時に暗くされてもね£.
なかなか寝れないなって, あろうかと思うんですが : ,
う : : ん. おそらく, 避けた方がいいと思います.

113 P I see.
はい.
[00:09:15]

114 P Well, it will be getting warmer soon.
まあ, もうちょっとで温かくなってきますからね.

115 D Yes.
う : : ん.

116 P What will happen then[?
それでどうなる[か.

117 D [What will happen?
The swelling in your feet and all that should be fine.
[どうなるか.
足元むくんだりとかは, 大丈夫でしょうかね.

118 N Let's get you on the scale.
ちょっと体重計に.

119 P ((moving onto the scale))
(27.0)

120 N Okay. All done.
はい (.) いいですよ.

121 P But, thanks to you, it's getting much better.
でもね, おかげさまでだいぶ良くなったんで,

122 D Yes, the movement of your back has gotten much better.
うん. 腰がね, 動きが, シャンとされましたね.

123	P	Yes. ええ. (30.0) ((setting back, writing and checking for scheduling))
124	D	Did I give you our schedule for April? ((contractual part)) 4月の予定表ってお渡ししたんでしたっけ ↑
125	P	Yes, I have it already. あ (.) もうあります. (14.0)
126	D	Today I'll give you medicine- a prescription for enough to last until the 23rd. <不足しにくいように>,ちょっとお薬を, 23の分まで足りるように, 今日はお薬を- 処方箋をお出ししておきますから,
127	P	Yes, yes. はいはい.
128	D	Please get these ready, okay? And the ointment for your skin, too, I'll prescribe it today so you don't run out. お願いして, 貰っておいてもらいましょうね. あとその, お肌塗る薬とかも, 今日不足しないように, 出しておきましょうね.
129	P	Okay. About the medicines, after I get them, I leave everything up to the staff. はい (.) 薬はあの, 頂いたやつをそっくりそのまま預けちゃうんですよ.
130	D	Right, right. ええ, ええ.
131	P	They manage it for me, and, 向こうでなんか管理してて,
132	D	Right. Well, はい. え : : っと,
133	P	then, they bring it with each meal three times a day. で, 3食, 食事の時, 持ってきてくれて.
134	D	Today, I'll give you the same tablets as usual and ointment, the compress and eye drops, and, um, you're also [drinking one can of Enshua, right? 今日はいつもの飲み薬と, 塗るやつと, 湿布と目薬と, え : : と, エンシュアって缶のやつも一つ[のんでますね↑
135	P	I am. [飲んでます.
136	D	Okay. [With that, はい. それも合わせ[て,
137	P	[I divide it into two parts per day. [2回に分けて一日に.
138	D	Ah, you've got to make sure you're getting enough nutrition. あ, ぜひしっかり, 栄養も取らないとね=

139 P Yes.
はい.
140 D You've got to. Okay, then, I'll give you your prescriptions for today. Please get them.
((getting ready for the off))
=いけませんからね.
それでじゃあ, 今日は処方箋をお渡ししておきます.
これをね, お願いして貰ってください.
(7.0)
[00:12:14]
141 D If your pain continues to be better for a while longer,
I think we could <u>probably</u> try to reduce the amount of the painkiller, [but,
もうちょっと痛みが, 落ち着いてる状態が続けば,
痛み止めを少し減らしてみても<u>いいかな</u>とも思っているんです[けど.
142 P I see.
[そうですね.
143 D Yes.
ええ, ええ.
144 P Let's see how it goes for one more visit.
もう一回くらい, 様子みましょう.
145 D Right. Let's see how it goes.
Things like your back pain might change when it gets warmer, too. We can make a decision while seeing how things go.
そうですね. ちょっと様子見ましょう.
で, また温かくなると, またね腰とか色々変わるかもしれませんし,
ちょっと様子をみながら判断しましょうか.
146 P Yes. Thank you.
はい (.) よろしくお願いします.
147 D Alright, for April, our next visit is scheduled for the 2nd.
So our next visit is 2nd April. See you then.
((closing the session))
あとですね, 4月, 次回2日を予定しています.
次回4月2日ですね. そこでまたお会いしましょう.
148 P Okay.
そうですね.
149 D And, um, as a result of the fiscal year changing over in April, I'll have to be in the clinic to see outpatients, rather than doing home visits. From April onwards, your visiting <doctor> will [change from me to another doctor.
で, あの : : 4月から年度が変わるのに合わせて,
ちょっと, 私この時間帯ですね, 往診じゃなくて,
外来, いらっしゃる方の診療の方にでないといけないので,
4月からは伺う<医師>が,
担当の医師が, 私からちょっと他の医師に[交代になります.
150 P [Right. I understand.
[はいはい. そうですか.

151 D But for the visit on 2nd April, I'll [come] with.
Take care until then.
ただ, 4月2日の日は, とりあえず一緒に[伺いますので,]
またどうぞ宜しくお願い[いたしますどうぞ.]
152 P [Right, right.]
[はいはい.]
[00:13:26]
153 D Do you have any concerns? Is everything okay?
((asks P's son))
息子さん何か, 気になってらっしゃることとか. 大丈夫ですか↑
154 PF-S It's fine.
大丈夫ですね.
155 D Sounds like everything's okay.
特になさそうですね.
156 PF-S So, it won't be you anymore.
先生じゃなくなっちゃうんですね.
157 D I'll be in the clinic, but not for home visits,
いるにはいるんですが, 往診に伺うの[が,
158 PF-S [Just home visits.
[往診は.
159 D Yes, yes.
はいはい.
160 P Doctor, I have one concern,
((topic initiation))
先生一つね, 気になってるのですが,
161 D Yes, yes. What is it?
はいはい (.) なんでしょう↑
162 P My hearing has gotten quite poor.
だいぶ耳が遠くなってきたんですよ.
163 D Right, right, right.
ええ : ええ : ええ : .
164 P Should I just let it be?
Or, is it better to see a specialist?
これ放っておいていいかしら.
それとも医者行ったほうがいい↑
165 D Um. Well, I remember that you went to see an otolaryngologist before.
う : ん (.) あの以前に,
耳鼻科の方で診てもらったことも確かあって,
166 P Yes, yes.
はいはい.
167 D Well, I don't think it's a sign of a particular illness
or anything like that.
あの : : 特別な病気の兆候とか,
そういったことは (.) ないと思うんです.
168 P Ah, I see.
あ (.) そうですか.
169 D Yes, and,
うん : [で,

170	P	[Maybe, because of ageing… [年齢からくるあれかしらね.
171	D	Yes. And if you would like treatment, it wouldn't be with medicine or an operation but, the use of a hearing aid, はい. で, 対処するんであれば, 特別な薬とか, 手術とかではなくて, ま, 補聴器とかを使って,
172	P	Ah.
173	D	in order to be able to hear. [I would think. 聞こえるようにするっていう形になると[思うんですね.
174	P	[Ah, I see.] Okay. [あ, そうですか.] はい.
175	D	Hearing aids are expensive, and surprisingly difficult to put in. They also make unwanted noises louder, 補聴器も値段がするのと, あと付けるのが意外と億劫だったり, 雑音も大きくなるのでうるさかったり,
176	P	I see. ええ.
177	D	because of that, there are some people for whom they aren't suitable. If it's bothering you, I recommend that you see an otolaryngologist [rather] than going to a shop for a hearing aid. <Otolaryngologists> can explain which one is better for you to buy after an examination. そういうので合わない方もいらっしゃるので, お困りなようだったら, 一回耳鼻科に行くと, その補聴器のどういったのがいいよって, 紹介もしてくれたりしますから, 補聴器屋さんに行くよりは, 耳鼻科の<お医者さん>に診てもらった上で紹介して[もらったほうが=]
178	P	Ah, I see. [あ : : そうですか.]
179	D	I think that's better. =いいと思いますけど.
180	P	Yes. はい.
181	D	Right. う : : ん.
182	P	Thank you very much. ありがとうございます.
183	D	I think it's very difficult to cure. なかなか, 治すっていうのは, 難しいかと思いますね.
184	P	I see, for ears. Yes. Thank you very much. そうですね, 耳はね. はい, ありがとうございました.
185	D	Then, if you'll excuse me, I'll see you <in two weeks>. ((concluding the conversation)) じゃあすみませんが, また<2週間後>かな,
186	PF-S	Right. そうですね.

187	D	See you next time. ((heading for the entrance)) また伺います.
188	N	Right. Then, see you next time. はい (.) じゃあ失礼しま：す.

Note

(1) The authors adapt a number of diagnostics models on clinical problem-solving and questioning skills that address specific disease types and/or status into Japanese primary care settings: for example, the Saint-Frances Guide to Outpatient Medicine (Frances *et al.*, 2000); A clinically relevant classification of chest discomfort (Diamond, 1983); Case-finding instruments for depression: two questions are as good as many (Whooley *et al.*, 1997).

References

Agency of Cultural Affairs, Governments of Japan (2007) Keigo no Shishin [Guidelines on honorific expressions]. See http://www.bunka.go.jp/seisaku/bunkashingikai/kokugo/hokoku/pdf/keigo_tosin.pdf (accessed 28 June 2021) [in Japanese].

Ammentorp, J., Graugaard, L.T., Lau, M.E., Andersen, T.P., Waidtlow, K. and Kofoed, P.E. (2014) Mandatory communication training of all employees with patient contact. *Patient Education and Counseling* 95 (3), 429–432.

Atkins, S., Roberts, C., Hawthorne, K. and Greenhalgh, T. (2016) Simulated consultations: A sociolinguistic perspective. *BMC Medical Education* 16 (1), 16.

Backhaus, P. (2009) Politeness in institutional elderly care in Japan: A cross-cultural comparison. *Journal of Politeness Research* 5, 3–71.

Backhaus, P. (2017) *Care Communication: Making a Home in a Japanese Eldercare Facility*. Abingdon: Routledge.

Balint, M., Hunt, J., Joyce, D., Marinker, M. and Woodcock, J. (1970) *Treatment or Diagnosis: A Study of Repeat Prescriptions in General Practice*. Toronto, OT: J.B. Lippincott.

Barello, S. and Graffigna, G. (2020) Caring for health professionals in the COVID-19 pandemic emergency: Toward an "epidemic of empathy" in Healthcare. *Frontiers in Psychology* 11, 1–4.

Brown, J. (2008) How clinical communication has become a core part of medical education in the UK. *Medical Education* 42 (3), 271–278.

Brown, J., Noble, L., Papageorgiou, A. and Kidd, J. (eds) (2016) *Clinical Communication in Medicine*. Chichester: Wiley Blackwell.

Brown, P. and Levinson, S.C. (1987) *Politeness: Some Universals in Language Usage*. Cambridge: Cambridge University Press.

Brugel, S., Postma-Nilsenova, M. and Tates, K. (2015) The link between perception of clinical empathy and nonverbal behavior: The effect of a doctor's gaze and body orientation. *Patient Education and Counseling* 98 (10), 1260–1265.

Buckman, R. (2000) *How to Break Bad News: A Guide for Health Care Professionals* (Japanese edn, S. Tsuneto trans.). Tokyo: Shindan To Chiryo Sha [in Japanese].

Byrne, P.S. and Long, B.E.L. (1984) *Doctors Talking to Patients: A Study of the Verbal Behaviour of General Practitioners Consulting in Their Surgeries*. Exeter: Royal College of General Practitioners.

Cabinet Office Government of Japan (2018) Annual report on the aging society [summary], health and welfare services for the elderly. See https://www8.cao.go.jp/kourei/whitepaper/index-w.html (accessed 28 June 2021).

Caldwell, J.G. (2008) Evaluating attitudes of first-year residents to shared decision making. *Medical Education Online* 13 (1), 1–6.

Cegala, D.J. and Post, D.M. (2009) The impact of patients' participation on physicians' patient-centered communication. *Patient Education and Counseling* 77 (2), 202–208.

Cole, S.A. and Bird, J. (1994) *The Medical Interview: The Three-Function Approach* (Japanese edn, K. Iijima and M. Sasaki trans.). Tokyo: Medical Sciences International [in Japanese].

Cole, S.A. and Bird, J. (2014) *The Medical Interview: The Three Function Approach* (3rd edn). Philadelphia, PA: Saunders.

Common Achievement Tests Organization (2020) Common achievement tests for medical and dental students prior to clinical clerkship. See http://www.cato.umin.jp/osce.html (accessed 28 June 2021) [in Japanese].

Cook, H.M. (2011) Are honorifics polite? Uses of referent honorifics in a Japanese committee meeting. *Journal of Pragmatics* 43, 3655–3672.

Crezee, I. and Asano, T. (2016) *Introduction to Healthcare for Japanese-speaking Interpreters and Translators*. Amsterdam: John Benjamins.

Diamond, G.A. (1983) A clinically relevant classification of chest discomfort. *Journal of the American College of Cardiology* 1 (2 Part 1), 574–575.

Eelen, G. (2001) *A Critique of Politeness Theories*. Manchester: St Jerome Publishing.

Eklund, J.H., Holmstrom, I.K., Kumlin, T., Kaminsky, E., Skoglund, K., Hoglander, J., Sundler, A.J., Conden, E. and Meranius, M.S. (2019) "Same same or different?" A review of reviews of person-centered and patient-centered care. *Patient Education and Counseling* 102 (1), 3–11.

Epstein, R.M. (1999) Mindful practice. *The Journal of The American Medical Association* 9, 833.

Epstein, R.M. (2003) Mindful practice in action (I): Technical competence, evidence-based medicine, and relationship-centered care. *Families, Systems & Health* 21 (1), 1.

Epstein, R.M. and Street, R.L. (2007) Patient-centered communication in cancer care: Promoting healing and reducing suffering. *National Cancer Institute, U.S. Department of Health and Human Services*. No. 07-6225.

Epstein, R.M., Morse, D., Frankel, R., Frarey, L., Anderson, K. and Beckman, H. (1998) Awkward moments in patient-physician communication about HIV risk. *Annals of Internal Medicine* 128 (6), 435–442.

Epstein, R.M., Franks, P., Fiscella, K., Shields, C., Meldrum, S., Kravitz, R. and Duberstein, P. (2005) Measuring patient-centered communication in patient–physician consultations: Theoretical and practical issues. *Social Science & Medicine* 61, 1516–1528.

Finset, A., Bosworth, H., Butow, P., Gulbrandsen, P., Hulsman, R.L., Pieterse, A.H., Street, R., Tschoetschel, R. and van Weert, J. (2020) Effective health communication – A key factor in fighting the COVID-19 pandemic. *Patient Education and Counseling* 103 (5), 873.

Frances, C., Bent, S. and Saint, S. (2000) *Saint-Frances Guide to Outpatient Medicine* (3rd edn). Philadelphia, PA: Lippincott Williams & Wilkins.

Fujisaki, K. (1997) *Medical Sociology [Wakariyasui Iryo-shakai-gaku]*. Tokyo: Kango no Kagaku Sha [in Japanese].

Fujisaki, K., Kawakami, C., Kato, T. and Takahashi, Y. (2015) *Mogi-shinsatsu Shinario-shu [Roll Play Scenario for Medical Interviews]*. Nagoya: Sankeisha [in Japanese].

Fukada, A. and Asato, N. (2004) Universal politeness theory: Application to the use of Japanese honorifics. *Journal of Pragmatics* 36, 1991–2002.

Fukushima, S. (2000) *Requests and Culture: Politeness in British English and Japanese*. Bern: Peter Lang.

Goetz, J.L., Keltner, D. and Simon-Thomas, E. (2010) Compassion: An evolutionary analysis and empirical review. *Psychological Bulletin* 136 (3), 351–374.

Goffman, E. (1967) *Interaction Ritual: Essays on Face-To-Face Behaviour*. New York: Doubleday Anchor.

Golato, A. (2003) Studying compliment responses: A comparison of DCTs and recordings of naturally occurring talk. *Applied Linguistics* 24 (1), 90–121.

Gold, R.L. (1958) Roles in sociological field observation. *Social Forces* 36, 217–223.

Goldberg, D.P., Steele, J.L., Smith, C. and Spivey, L. (1983) *Training Family Practice Residents to Recognise Psychiatric Disturbances*. Rockville, MD: National Institute of Mental Health.

Grainger, K. (2004) Communication and the institutionalized elderly. In J.F. Nussbaum and J. Coupland (eds) *Handbook of Communication and Aging Research* (2nd edn, pp. 740–775) London: Laurence Erlbaum Associates.
Green, J. and Thorogood, N. (2018) *Qualitative Methods for Health Research*. London: Sage.
Greenhill, N., Anderson, C., Avery, A. and Pilnick, A. (2011) Analysis of pharmacist–patient communication using the Calgary-Cambridge guide. *Patient Education and Counseling* 83 (3), 423–431.
Gu, Y. (1990) Politeness phenomena in modern Chinese. *Journal of Pragmatics* 14 (2), 237–257.
Gudykunst, W.B., Matsumoto, Y., Ting-Toomey, S., Nishida, T., Kim, I. and Heyman, S. (1996) The influence of cultural individualism-collectivism, self construals, and individual values on communication styles across cultures. *Human Communication Research* 22, 510–543.
Hall, E. and Hall, M. (1990) *Understanding Cultural Differences: Germans, French and Americans*. Yarmouth: Intercultural Press.
Hall, E.T. (1976) *Beyond Culture*. New York: Doubleday.
Hammersley, M. (1992) Some reflections on ethnography and validity. *Qualitative Studies in Education* 5 (3), 195–203.
Hammond, M. and McLean, E. (2009) What parents and carers think medical students should be learning about communication with children and families. *Patient Education and Counseling* 76 (3), 368–375.
Haugh, M. (2007) The discursive challenge to politeness research: An interactional alternative. *Journal of Politeness Research* 3 (2), 295–317.
Hepburn, A. and Bolden, G.B. (2013) The conversation analytic approach to transcription. In J. Sidnell and T. Stivers (eds) *Blackwell Handbook of Conversation Analysis* (pp. 57–76). Oxford: Blackwell.
Hilder, J., Gray, B. and Stubbe, M. (2019) Integrating health navigation and interpreting services for patients with limited English proficiency: Views of Pacific navigators. *Pacific Health Dialog* 21 (3), 116–127.
Hirota, N. (1992) *"Ishi no Tachiba kara" [From the Viewpoint of a Physician]* (pp. 192–193). Ureshino: Ureshino National Hospital [in Japanese].
Hofstede, G. (1984) *Culture's Consequences: International Differences in Work-Related Values*. Beverly Hills, CA: SAGE.
Hofstede, G. (1991) *Cultures and Organizations: Software of the Mind*. London: McGraw-Hill.
Hofstede, G., Hofstede, G.J. and Minkov, M. ([1991] 2010) *Cultures and Organizations: Software of the Mind* (3rd edn). London: McGraw-Hill.
Hojat, M. (2007) *Empathy in Patient Care: Antecedents, Development, Measurement and Outcomes*. New York: Springer.
Hojat, M., Mangione, S., Nasca, T.J., Cohen, M.J., Gonnella, J.S., Erdmann, J.B., Veloski, J. and Magee, M. (2001) The Jefferson Scale of Physician Empathy: Development and preliminary psychometric data. *Educational and Psychological Measurement* 61 (2), 349–365.
Hojat, M., Gonnella, J.S., Mangione, S., Nasca, T.J., Veloski, J.J., Erdmann, J.B., Callahan, C.A. and Magee, M. (2002) Empathy in medical students as related to academic performance, clinical competence and gender. *Medical Education* 36 (6), 522–527.
Hojat, M., Vergare, M., Isenberg, G., Cohen, M. and Spandorfer, J. (2015) Underlying construct of empathy, optimism, and burnout in medical students. *International Journal of Medical Education* 6, 12–16.
Holmes, J. and Stubbe, M. (2015) *Power and Politeness in the Workplace: A Sociolinguistic Analysis of Talk at Work* (2nd edn). Abingdon: Routledge.
Holt, G.R. (2020) The pandemic effect: Raising the bar for ethics, empathy, and professional collegiality. *Otolaryngology Head and Neck Surgery* 163 (4), 621–622.

Holtgraves, T. (2005) Social psychology, cognitive psychology, and linguistic politeness. *Journal of Politeness Research: Language, Behavior, Culture* 1, 73–93.

Houchens, N. and Tipirneni, R. (2020) Compassionate communication amid the COVID-19 pandemic. *Journal of Hospital Medicine* 15 (7), 437–439.

Howie, J.G., Heaney, D. and Maxwell, M. (2004) Quality, core values and the general practice consultation: Issues of definition, measurement and delivery. *Family Practice* 21, 458–468.

Ide, S. (1989) Formal forms and discernment: Two neglected aspects of universals of linguistic politeness. *Multilingua Journal of Cross-cultural and Interlanguage Communication* 8, 223–248.

Ide, S., Hill, B., Carnes, Y.M., Ogino, T. and Kawasaki, A. (1992) The concept of politeness: An empirical study of American English and Japanese. In R. Watts, S. Ide and K. Ehlich (eds) *Politeness in Language: Studies in Its History, Theory and Practice* (pp. 281–298). Berlin: Mouton de Gruyter.

Ikuta, S. (1983) Speech level shift and conversational strategy in Japanese discourse. *Language Sciences* 5, 37–53.

Inoue, I. (1997) Menmoku Saikou: Ibunka-Communication no Kanten kara [Face Reconsideration from the perspective of Intercultural Communication]. *Jinbun-Kagaku Ronshu* 31, 67–82 [in Japanese].

Ishikawa, H. and Yamazaki, Y. (2005) How applicable are western models of patient-physician relationship in Asia?: Changing patient-physician relationship in contemporary Japan. *International Journal of Japanese Sociology* 14, 84–93.

Ishikawa, H., Takayama, T., Yamazaki, Y., Seki, Y. and Katsumata, N. (2002) Physician-patient communication and patient satisfaction in Japanese cancer consultations. *Social Science and Medicine* 55, 301–311.

Ishikawa, H., Eto, M, Kitamura, K. and Kiuchi, T. (2014) Resident physicians' attitudes and confidence in communicating with patients: A pilot study at a Japanese university hospital. *Patient Education & Counseling* 96 (3), 361–366.

Ishikawa, H., Son, D., Eto, M., Kitamura, K. and Kiuchi, T. (2018) Changes in patient-centered attitude and confidence in communicating with patients: A longitudinal study of resident physicians. *BMC Medical Education* 18 (1), 20.

Jefferson, G. (2004) Glossary of transcript symbols with an introduction. In G.H. Lerner (ed.) *Conversation Analysis: Studies from the First Generation* (pp. 13–31). Amsterdam: John Benjamins.

Jeffrey, D. (2016) Empathy, sympathy and compassion in healthcare: Is there a problem? Is there a difference? Does it matter? *Journal of the Royal Society of Medicine* 109 (12), 446–452.

Kadar, D.Z. and Haugh, M. (2013) *Understanding Politeness*. Cambridge: Cambridge University Press.

Kalet, A., Pugnaire, M., Cole-Kelly, K., Janicik, R., Ferrara, E., Schwartz, M., Lipkin, M. and Lazare, A. (2004) Teaching communication in clinical clerkships: Models from the Macy Initiative in Health Communications. *Academic Medicine: Journal of The Association of American Medical Colleges* 79 (6), 511–520.

Kasper, G. (1990) Linguistic politeness: Current research issues. *Journal of Pragmatics* 14 (2), 193–218.

Kasper, G. (2000) Data collection in pragmatics research. In H. Spencer-Oatey (ed.) *Culturally Speaking: Managing Rapport Through Talk Across Cultures* (pp. 316–341). London: Continuum.

Kasper, G. and Dahl, M. (1991) Research methods in interlanguage pragmatics. *Studies in Second Language Acquisition* 13 (2), 215–247.

Kataoka, H.U., Koide, N., Ochi K, Hojat, M. and Gonnella, J.S. (2009) Measurement of empathy among Japanese medical students: Psychometrics and score differences by gender and level of medical education. *Academic Medicine* 84, 1192–1197.

Katsuno, T. (2005) Dementia from the inside: How people with early-stage dementia evaluate their quality of life. *Ageing & Society* 25 (2), 197–214.

Kelly, S. (2010) Qualitative interviewing techniques and styles. In I. Bourgeault, R. Dingwall and R. De Vries (eds) *The SAGE Handbook of Qualitative Methods in Health Research* (pp. 307–326). London: SAGE.
Kirschenbaum, H. and Jourdan, A. (2005) The current status of carl rogers and the person-centered approach. *Psychotherapy: Theory, Research, Practice, Training* 42 (1), 37–51.
Kisa, K., Kawabata, H., Itou, T., Nishimoto, N. and Maezawa, M. (2011) Survey of patient and physician satisfaction regarding patient-centered outpatient consultations in Japan. *Internal Medicine* 50 (13), 1403–1408.
Kita, S. and Ide, S. (2009) Nodding, aizuchi, and final particles in Japanese conversation: How conversation reflects the ideology of communication and social relationships. *Journal of Pragmatics* 39 (7), 1242–1254.
Kittler, M.G., Rygl, D. and Mackinnon, A. (2011) Special review article: Beyond culture or beyond control? Reviewing the use of Hall's high-/low-context concept. *International Journal of Cross Cultural Management* 11 (1), 63–82.
Koizumi, S. (2010) General medicine and health professions education. *An Official Journal of the Japan Primary Care Association* 33 (4), 431–436.
Kuga, S., Kachi, Y., Inoue, M. and Kawada, T. (2016) Characteristics of general physicians who practice shared decision making: A mail survey of all clinics in 12 municipalities in Tokyo. *Japan Primary Care Association* 39 (4), 209–213 [in Japanese].
Kurtz, S., Silverman, J., Benson, J. and Draper, J. (2003) Marrying content and process in clinical method teaching: Enhancing the Calgary-Cambridge guides. *Academic Medicine* 78, 802–809.
Lambert, B.L. (1996) Face and politeness in pharmacist-physician interaction. *Social Science & Medicine* 43 (8), 1189–1198.
Lanceley, A. (1985) Use of controlling language in the rehabilitation of the elderly. *Journal of Advanced Nursing* 10, 125–135.
Lawrence, E.J., Shaw, P., Baker, D., Baron-Cohen, S. and David, A.S. (2004) Measuring empathy: Reliability and validity of the empathy quotient. *Psychological Medicine* 34 (5), 911–919.
Legare, F. and Witteman, H.O. (2013) Shared decision making: Examining key elements and barriers to adoption into routine clinical practice. *Health Affairs* 32 (2), 276–284.
Levenstein, J.H., Brown, J.B., Weston, W.W., Stewart, M., McCracken, E.C. and McWhinney, I. (1989) Patient-centered clinical interviewing. In M. Stewart and D. Roter (eds) *Communicating with Medical Patients* (pp. 107–120). London: Sage Publications.
Liu, S., Volcic, Z. and Gallois, C. (2011) *Introducing Intercultural Communication: Global Cultures and Contexts*. London: SAGE.
Locher, M.A. (2006) Polite behavior within relational work: The discursive approach to politeness. *Multilingua* 25 (3), 249–267.
Locher, M.A. (2015) Interpersonal pragmatics and its link to (im)politeness research. *Journal of Pragmatics* 86, 5–10.
Locher, M.A. (2017) *Reflective Writing in Medical Practice: A Linguistic Perspective*. Bristol: Multilingual Matters.
Locher, M.A. and Schnurr, S. (2017) (Im)politeness in health settings. In J. Culpeper, M. Haugh and D. Kadar (eds) *The Palgrave Handbook of Linguistic (Im)politeness* (pp. 689–711). London: Palgrave Macmillan.
Locher, M.A. and Watts, R.J. (2005) Politeness theory and relational work. *Journal of Politeness Research* 1 (1), 9–33.
Maeda, I. (2005) *Jissen, Kanja Manzoku-do Up [Patient Satisfaction]*. Tokyo: Nihon Hyoron-sha [in Japanese].
Makoni, S. and Grainger, K. (2002) Comparative gerontolinguistics: Characterizing discourses in caring institutions in South Africa and the United Kingdom. *Journal of Social Issues* 58, 805–824.

Mao, L.R. (1994) Beyond politeness theory: 'Face' revisited and renewed. *Journal of Pragmatics* 21, 451–486.

Matsumoto, Y. (1988) Reexamination of the universality of face: Politeness phenomena in Japanese. *Journal of Pragmatics* 12, 403–426.

Matsumura, S. and Minowa, Y. (2007) *Communication Skill Training, Customer Satisfaction Training*. Tokyo: Igaku-Shoin [in Japanese].

Matsushige, T. (2010) *The Discourse of 'Patient-Centred Medicine': The Sociology of Patient Expertise*. Tokyo: Rikkyo University Press [in Japanese].

Matusitz, J. and Spear, J. (2015) Doctor-patient communication styles: A comparison between the United States and three Asian countries. *Journal of Human Behavior in the Social Environment* 25, 871–884.

Maynard, S. (1993) *Kaiwabunseki [Conversational Analysis]*. Tokyo: Kuroshio [in Japanese].

McCormack, B. (2003) A conceptual framework for person-centred practice with older people. *International Journal of Nursing Practice* 3, 202.

McCormack, L.A., Treiman, K., Rupert, D., Williams-Piehota, P., Nadler, E., Arora, N.K., Lawrence, W. and Street, R.L. (2011) Measuring patient-centered communication in cancer care: A literature review and the development of a systematic approach. *Social Science & Medicine* 72, 1085–1095.

McKinstry, B. (1992) Paternalism and the doctor-patient relationship in general practice. *British Journal of General Practice* 42 (361), 340–342.

McKinstry, B. (2000) Do patients wish to be involved in decision making in the consultation? A cross sectional survey with video vignettes. *BMJ (Clinical Research Ed.)* 321 (7265), 867–871.

McWhinney, I. (1989) The need for a transformed clinical method. In M. Stewart and D. Roter (eds) *Communicating with Medical Patients* (pp. 25–42). London: Sage.

Mead, N. and Bower, P. (2000) Patient-centredness: A conceptual framework and review of the empirical literature. *Social Science & Medicine* 51, 1087–1110.

Mills, S. (2011) Discursive approaches to politeness and impoliteness. In Linguistic Politeness Research Group (eds) *Discursive Approaches to Politeness* (pp. 19–56). Berlin: de Gruyter Mouton.

Ministry of Health, Labour and Welfare (2016) Long-term care insurance system of Japan: Procedure for use of long-term care services (p. 10). See http://www.mhlw.go.jp/english/policy/care-welfare/care-welfare-elderly/dl/ltcisj_e.pdf (accessed 28 June 2021).

Miyata, Y. and Mukohara, K. (2015) Joint principles for the medical education of physicians as preparation for practice in the patient-centered medical home. *The Japanese Society of Internal Medicine* 104 (2), 340–349.

Mondaca, M., Josephsson, S., Katz, A. and Rosenberg, L. (2018) Influencing everyday activities in a nursing home setting: A call for ethical and responsive engagement. *Nursing Inquiry* 25 (2), e12217.

Morand, D.A. (1996) Dominance, deference, and egalitarianism in organizational interaction: A sociolinguistic analysis of power and politeness. *Organization Science* 7, 544–556.

Morand, D.A. (2000) Language and power: An empirical analysis of linguistic strategies used in superior-subordinate communication. *Journal of Organizational Behavior* 21, 235–248.

Morand, D.A. (2003) Politeness and the clash of interaction orders in cross-cultural communication. *Thunderbird International Business Review* 45, 521–540.

Moss, B. and Roberts, C. (2005) Explanations, explanations, explanations: How do patients with limited English construct narrative accounts in multi-lingual, multi-ethnic settings, and how can GPs interpret them? *Family Practice* 22 (4), 412–418.

Mukohara, K. (2006) *Medical Interview: Evidence-Based Approach*. Tokyo: Bunkyo-Do [in Japanese].

Mullany, L. (2009) Introduction: Applying politeness research to health care communication. *Journal of Politeness Research: Language, Behavior, Culture* 5, 1–10.

Musolff, A., Breeze, R., Kondo, K. and Vilar-Lluch, S. (eds) (2022) *Pandemic and Crisis Discourse: Communicating COVID-19 and Public Health Strategy*. London: Bloomsbury Publishing.

Nikendei, C., Bosse, H.M., Hoffmann, K., Moltner, A., Hancke, R., Conrad, C. and Schultz, J.H. (2011) Outcome of parent–physician communication skills training for pediatric residents. *Patient Education and Counseling* 82 (1), 94–99.

Noguchi, Y. and Fukuhara, S. (2008) *Daremo oshiete-kurenakatta Shindan Gaku [No one taught me Diagnostic Science]*. Tokyo: Igaku-Shoin.

Norris, P. and Rowsell, B. (2003) Interactional issues in the provision of counselling to pharmacy customers. *International Journal of Pharmacy Practice* 11 (3), 135–142.

Northouse, L. and Northouse, P. (1997) *Health Communication: Strategies for Health Professionals*. Connecticut: Appleton and Lange.

Ohtaki, S., Ohtaki, T. and Fetters, M.D. (2003) Doctor–patient communication: A comparison of the USA and Japan. *Family Practice* 20, 276–282.

Okushi, Y. (1988) Use of Japanese Honorifics in daily life: What the traditional theories do not say. *ERIC*, ED422716. See https://eric.ed.gov/?id=ED422716.

Okutani, T., Hamada, H., Batty, H.P. and Otani, T. (2007) A new trend toward interprofessional education in Canada. *Medical Education* 38 (3), 181–185.

Ordóñez-López, P. and Edo-Marzá, N. (eds) (2016) *Medical Discourse in Professional, Academic and Popular Settings*. Bristol: Multilingual Matters.

Ottrey, E., Palermo, C., Huggins, C.E. and Porter, J. (2020) A longitudinal ethnographic study of hospital staff attitudes and experiences of change in nutrition care. *Journal of Human Nutrition and Dietetics* 33 (4), 574–583.

Ouwens, M., Hermens, R., Hulscher, M., Vonk-Okhuijsen, S., Tjan-Heijnen, V., Termeer, R., Marres, H., Wollersheim, H. and Grol, R. (2010) Development of indicators for patient-centred cancer care. *Supportive Care in Cancer: Official Journal of The Multinational Association of Supportive Care in Cancer* 18 (1), 121–130.

Oyserman, D., Coon, H. and Kemmelmeier, M. (2002) Rethinking individualism and collectivism: Evaluation of theoretical assumptions and meta-analyses. *Psychological Bulletin* 128, 3–72.

Pizziconi, B. (2003) Re-examining politeness, face and the Japanese language. *Journal of Pragmatics* 35, 1471–1506.

Potter, J. (2002) Two kinds of natural. *Discourse Studies* 4 (4), 539–542.

Pounds, G. (2011) Empathy as "appraisal": A new language-based approach to the exploration of clinical empathy. *Journal of Applied Linguistics and Professional Practice* 7 (2), 139–162.

Pounds, G. (2018) Patient-centred communication in ask-the-expert healthcare websites. *Applied Linguistics* 39 (2), 117–134.

Pounds, G. and De Pablos-Ortega, C. (2016) Patient-centred communication in British, Italian and Spanish ask-the-Expert healthcare websites. *Communication and Medicine* 12 (2–3), 225–241.

Pounds, G., Salter, C., Platt, M.J. and Bryant, P. (2018) Developing a new empathy-specific admissions test for applicants to medical schools: A discourse-pragmatic approach. *Communication and Medicine* 14 (2), 165–180.

Ramani, S., Konings, K.D., Mann, K.V., Pisarski, E.E. and van der Vleuten, C.P. (2018) About politeness, face, and feedback: Exploring resident and faculty perceptions of how institutional feedback culture influences feedback practices. *Academic Medicine* 93 (9), 1348–1358.

Roberts, C. (2009) Intercultural communication in healthcare settings. In H. Kotthoff and H. Spencer-Oatey (eds) *Handbook of Intercultural Communication* (pp. 243–262). New York: Mouton de Gruyter.

Roberts, C. and Moss, B. (Dir.) (2003) *Doing the Lambeth Talk* [Video/DVD]. King's College London. The DVD is available from the London Deanery, 20 Guild ford Street, London, WCIN 1DZ.

Roberts, C. and Sarangi, S. (2003) Uptake of discourse research in interprofessional settings: Reporting from medical consultancy. *Applied Linguistics* 24 (3), 338–359.

Roberts, C. and Sarangi, S. (2005) Theme-oriented discourse analysis of medical encounters. *Medical Education* 39 (6), 632–640.

Roberts, C., Sarangi, S. and Moss, R. (2004) Presentation of self and symptom in primary care consultations involving patients from non-English speaking backgrounds. *Communication & Medicine* 1 (2), 159–169.

Robins, L.S. and Wolf, F.M. (1988) Confrontation and politeness strategies in physician-patient interactions. *Social Science & Medicine* 27 (3), 217–221.

Rogers, C.R. ([1951] 2012) *Client-centered Therapy*. London: Robinson.

Rogers, C.R. ([1961] 1977) *On Becoming a Person: A Psychotherapists View of Psychotherapy*. London: Robinson.

Roter, D.L. and Hall, J.A. (2004) Physician gender and patient-centered communication: A critical review of empirical research. *Annual Review of Public Health* 25, 497–519.

Rudolf von Rohr, M.T., Thurnherr, F. and Locher, M.A. (2019) Linguistic expert creation in online health practices. In P. Bou-Franch and P. Garces-Conejos Blitvich (eds) *Analyzing Digital Discourse: New Insights and Future Directions* (pp. 219–250). Cham: Palgrave Macmillan.

Saito, S. (2000) *Hajimete no Iryo-mensetsu [Medical Interviews for Beginners]*. Tokyo: Igaku-Shoin [in Japanese].

Sarangi, S. (2005) The conditions and consequences of professional discourse studies. In R. Kiely, P. Rea-Dickens, H. Woodfield and G. Clibbon (eds) *Language, Culture and Identity in Applied Linguistics* (pp. 199–220). London: Equinox.

Sarangi, S. (2010a) Healthcare interaction as an expert communicative system: An activity analysis perspective. In J. Streeck (ed.) *New Adventures in Language and Interaction. Pragmatics & Beyond New Series* (pp. 167–197). Amsterdam: John Benjamins.

Sarangi, S. (2010b) Practising discourse analysis in healthcare settings. In I. Bourgeault, R. Dingwall and R. de Vries (eds) *The SAGE Handbook of Qualitative Methods in Health Research* (pp. 397–416). London: Sage.

Sarangi, S. and Roberts, C. (eds) (1999) *Talk, Work and Institutional Order: Discourse in Medical, Mediation and Management Settings*. Berlin: Mouton de Gruyter.

Scholl, I., Zill, J.M., Harter, M. and Dirmaier, J. (2014) An integrative model of patient-centeredness – A systematic review and concept analysis. *PLOS One* 9 (9), e107828.

Schwartz, S.H. (1992) Universals in the content and structure of values: Theoretical advances and empirical tests in 20 countries. *Advances in Experimental Social Psychology* 25, 1–65.

Schwartz, S.H. and Bardi, A. (2001) Value hierarchies across cultures. Take a similarities perspective. *Journal of Cross-Cultural Psychology* 32, 268–290.

Scollon, R., Scollon, S.W. and Jones, R.H. ([1995] 2011) *Intercultural Communication: A Discourse Approach* (3rd edn). Oxford: John Wiley & Sons, Inc.

Scott, J.G., Cohen, D., DiCicco-Bloom, B., Miller, W.L., Stange, K.C. and Crabtree, B.F. (2008) Understanding healing relationships in primary care. *The Annals of Family Medicine* 6 (4), 315–322.

Sharma, T., Bamford, M. and Dodman, D. (2015) Person-centred care: An overview of reviews. *Contemporary Nurse: A Journal for the Australian Nursing Profession* 51 (2–3), 107–120.

Shibamoto-Smith, J.S. (2011) Honorifics, politeness, and power in Japanese political debate. *Journal of Pragmatics* 43, 3707–3719.

Silverman, D. (2014) *Interpreting Qualitative Data* (4th edn). London: SAGE.

Silverman, J., Kurtz, S. and Draper, J. (2013) *Skills for Communicating with Patients* (3rd edn). London: Radcliffe Publishing.

Son, D., Shimizu, I., Ishikawa, H., Aomatsu, M. and Leppink, J. (2018) Communication skills training and the conceptual structure of empathy among medical students. *Perspectives on Medical Education* 7 (4), 264–271.

Soto-Rubio, A. and Sinclair, S. (2018) In defense of sympathy, in consideration of empathy, and in praise of compassion: A history of the present. *Journal of Pain and Symptom Management* 55 (5), 1428–1434.
Spencer-Oatey, H. (2007) Theories of identity and the analysis of face. *Journal of Pragmatics* 39 (4), 639–656.
Stewart, M., Brown, J., Weston, W., McWhinney, I., McWilliam, C. and Freeman, T. (1995) *Patient-Centered Medicine: Transforming the Clinical Method.* Thousand Oaks, CA: Sage Publications.
Stewart, M., Brown, J., Weston, W., McWhinney, I., McWilliam, C. and Freeman, T. ([1995] 2014) *Patient-Centered Medicine: Transforming the Clinical Method* (3rd edn). London: Redcliff Publishing Ltd.
Street, R.L. (2017) The many "disguises" of patient-centered communication: Problems of conceptualization and measurement. *Patient Education and Counseling* 100, 2131–2134.
Street, R.L. (1992) Analyzing communication in medical consultations: Do behavioral measures correspond to patients' perceptions? *Medical Care* 11, 976–988.
Suzuki, T. and Abe, K. (eds) (2011) *Yoku Wakaru Iryo-Mensetsu To Mogi-Kanja [Medical Interview and Simulated Patient].* Nagoya: University of Nagoya Press [in Japanese].
Takayama, T., Yamazaki, Y. and Katsumata, N. (2001) Relationship between outpatients' perceptions of physicians' communication styles and patients' anxiety levels in a Japanese oncology setting. *Social Science & Medicine* 53, 1335–1350.
Tannen, D. ([1984] 2005) *Conversational Style: Analyzing Talk Among Friends.* New York: Oxford University Press.
Taylor, K. (2009) Paternalism, participation and partnership—The evolution of patient centeredness in the consultation. *Patient Education and Counseling* 74 (2), 150–155.
Tokuda, Y., Yoshioka, Y., Aizawa, M., Tanaka, M., Ohde, S., Motomura, K., Naito, A., Hayano, K. and Fukui, T. (2008) Physicians' use of local dialects during communication with patients. *Journal of General and Family Medicine* 9, 13–19.
Triandis, H.C. (1989) The self and social behavior in different cultural contexts. *Psychological Review* 96, 269–289.
Triandis, H.C. (2001) Individualism-collectivism and personality. *Journal of Personality* 69 (6), 907–924.
Triandis, H.C., Bontempo, R., Betancourt, H., Bond, M., Leung, K., Brenes, A., Georgas, J., Hui, H., Martin, G., Setiadi, B., Sinha, J., Verma, J., Spangenberg, J., Touzard, H. and Montmollin, G. (1986) The measurement of the etic aspects of individualism and collectivism across cultures. *Australian Journal of Psychology* 38 (3), 257–267.
Uchida, H., Ota, A., Nagao, A., Yamawaki, N., Uemura, S., Tokuyama, C. and Mizutani, N. (1999) The difference of the cognition on informed consent between the citizens and the medical staff. *Japan Association for Bioethics* 9, 81–88 [in Japanese].
Usami, M. (1993) Sho-taimen no nisha-kan no kouzo to washa niyoru kaiwa no strategy [Communication strategy between unacquainted people]. *The Communication Association of Japan (CAJ)* 21, 25–40 [in Japanese].
Usami, M. (2002) *Discourse Politeness in Japanese Conversation: Some Implications for a Universal Theory of Politeness.* Tokyo: Hituzi Syobo.
Usami, M. (2008) Frontiers of studies on politeness theories: New trends in politeness studies and discourse politeness theory. *The Japanese Association of Sociolinguistic Sciences* 11, 4–22 [in Japanese].
Van Der Bom, I. and Grainger, K. (2015) Journal of politeness research: Introduction. *Journal of Politeness Research: Language, Behavior, Culture* 11, 165–178.
Van Der Bom, I. and Mills, S. (2015) A discursive approach to the analysis of politeness data. *Journal of Politeness Research* 11 (2), 179–206.

Van Dulmen, S. (2003) Editorial: Patient-centredness. *Patient Education and Counseling* 51, 195–196.

Vedel, M., Holma, A.M. and Havila, V. (2016) Conceptualizing inter-organizational triads. *Industrial Marketing Management* 57, 139–147.

Vilkki, L. (2006) Politeness, face and facework: Current issues. *SKY Journal of Linguistics* 19, 322–332.

Watanabe, S., Kodama, S. and Hanabusa, H. (2018) Longevity and elderly care: Lessons from Japan. *Global Health Journal* 2(4), 5–10.

Watts, R.J. (2003) *Politeness*. Cambridge: Cambridge University Press.

Whooley, M.A., Avins, A.L., Miranda, J. and Browner, W.S. (1997) Case-finding instruments for depression: Two questions are as good as many. *Journal of General Internal Medicine* 12 (7), 439–445.

Williams, G.C., McGregor, H., Zeldman, A., Freedman, Z.R., Deci, E.L. and Elder, D. (2005) Promoting glycemic control through diabetes self-management: Evaluating a patient activation intervention. *Patient Education and Counseling* 56, 28–34.

Wolff, J.L. and Roter, D.L. (2012) Older adults' mental health function and patient-centered care: Does the present of a family companion help or hinder communication? *Journal of General Internal Medicine* 27 (6), 661–668.

Wynn, R. and Wynn, M. (2006) Empathy as an interactionally achieved phenomenon in psychotherapy: Characteristics of some conversational resources. *Journal of Pragmatics* 38 (9), 1385–1397.

Yajima, R. and Takayanagi, K. (1998) The health care system: Citizen complaints, citizen possibilities. *Journal of Health and Human Services Administration* 20 (4), 502–519.

Yamaguchi, S., Cohen, S.R. and Uza, M. (2016) Family caregiving in Japan: The influence of cultural constructs in the care of adults with cancer. *Journal of Family Nursing* 22 (3), 392–418.

Yin, C.P., Hsu, C.W., Kuo, F.Y. and Huang, Y.T. (2012) A study of politeness strategies adopted in pediatric clinics in Taiwan. *Health Communication* 27 (6), 533–545.

Yoshioka, Y. and Shin, S. (2010) Clinical politeness strategy for appropriate communications between physicians and patients. *The Japanese Journal of Language in Society* 13, 35–47 [in Japanese].

Yoshioka, Y., Hayano, K., Tokuda, Y., Miura, J., Motomura, K., Aizawa, M., Tanaka, M. and Usami, M. (2008) Politeness strategy as an effective communication skill for improving the patient-physician relationship. *Igaku Kyoiku [Medical Education]* 39, 251–257 [in Japanese].

Zaleta, A.K. and Carpenter, B.D. (2010) Patient-centered communication during the disclosure of a dementia diagnosis. *American Journal of Alzheimer's Disease & Other Dementias* 25 (6), 513–520.

Author Index

Subject Index

For Product Safety Concerns and Information please contact our EU Authorised Representative:

Easy Access System Europe

Mustamäe tee 50

10621 Tallinn

Estonia

gpsr.requests@easproject.com

www.ingramcontent.com/pod-product-compliance
Ingram Content Group UK Ltd.
Pitfield, Milton Keynes, MK11 3LW, UK
UKHW021836150926
8656IPUK00003B/12